THE NLN JEFFRIES SIMULATION THEORY

SECOND EDITION

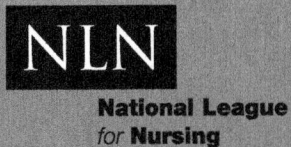

National League for Nursing

THE NLN JEFFRIES SIMULATION THEORY

SECOND EDITION

Edited by:
Pamela R. Jeffries, PhD, RN, FAAN, ANEF

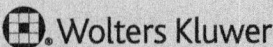

Philadelphia • Baltimore • New York • London
Buenos Aires • Hong Kong • Sydney • Tokyo

Vice President, Nursing Segment: Julie K. Stegman
Manager, Nursing Education and Practice Content: Jamie Blum
Senior Development Editor: Meredith L. Brittain
Marketing Manager: Greta H. Swanson
Editorial Assistant: Molly Kennedy
Manager, Graphic Arts and Design: Steve Druding
Senior Production Project Manager: David Saltzberg
Manufacturing Coordinator: Margie Orzech
Prepress Vendor: S4Carlisle Publishing Services

Copyright © 2022 National League for Nursing.

Jeffries, P. R. (2022). *The NLN Jeffries Simulation theory* (2nd ed.). National League for Nursing.

All rights reserved. This book is protected by copyright. No part of this book may be reproduced or transmitted in any form or by any means, including as photocopies or scanned-in or other electronic copies, or utilized by any information storage and retrieval system without written permission from the copyright owner, except for brief quotations embodied in critical articles and reviews. Materials appearing in this book prepared by individuals as part of their official duties as U.S. government employees are not covered by the previously mentioned copyright. To request permission, please contact Wolters Kluwer at Two Commerce Square, 2001 Market Street, Philadelphia, PA 19103, via email at permissions@lww.com, or via our website at shop.lww.com (products and services).

9 8 7 6 5 4 3 2 1

Printed in the United States of America

Library of Congress Cataloging-in-Publication Data

ISBN-13: 978-1-9751-8504-6
ISBN-10: 1-9751-8504-8
Library of Congress Control Number: 2021911327

Cataloging-in-Publication data available on request from the Publisher.

This work is provided "as is," and the publisher disclaims any and all warranties, express or implied, including any warranties as to accuracy, comprehensiveness, or currency of the content of this work.

This work is no substitute for individual patient assessment based upon healthcare professionals' examination of each patient and consideration of, among other things, age, weight, gender, current or prior medical conditions, medication history, laboratory data and other factors unique to the patient. The publisher does not provide medical advice or guidance and this work is merely a reference tool. Healthcare professionals, and not the publisher, are solely responsible for the use of this work including all medical judgments and for any resulting diagnosis and treatments.

Given continuous, rapid advances in medical science and health information, independent professional verification of medical diagnoses, indications, appropriate pharmaceutical selections and dosages, and treatment options should be made and healthcare professionals should consult a variety of sources. When prescribing medication, healthcare professionals are advised to consult the product information sheet (the manufacturer's package insert) accompanying each drug to verify, among other things, conditions of use, warnings and side effects and identify any changes in dosage schedule or contraindications, particularly if the medication to be administered is new, infrequently used or has a narrow therapeutic range. To the maximum extent permitted under applicable law, no responsibility is assumed by the publisher for any injury and/or damage to persons or property, as a matter of products liability, negligence law or otherwise, or from any reference to or use by any person of this work.

shop.lww.com   www.NLN.org

About the Editor

Pamela R. Jeffries, PhD, RN, FAAN, ANEF, an internationally recognized leader and innovator in nursing and health care education, is dean of the Vanderbilt University School of Nursing. In addition to her leadership, Dr. Jeffries is renowned for her strong expertise in experiential learning, innovative teaching strategies, new pedagogies, and the delivery of content using technology in nursing education. With support from the National League of Nursing (NLN), she developed the major contribution to simulation scholarship — the framework and monograph now known as the NLN Jeffries Simulation theory. A prolific collaborator, she is the editor of three other books, *Simulations in Nursing Education: From Conceptualization to Evaluation* (2nd edition), *Developing Simulation Centers Using the Consortium Model*, and *Clinical Simulations in Nursing Education: Advanced Concepts, Trends, and Opportunities*. 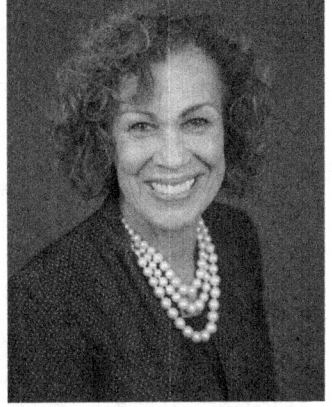 Throughout her career, she has been the recipient of several honors including the Sigma Theta Tau International Edith Moore Copeland Award for Excellence in Creativity, the NLN's Mary Adelaide Nutting Award for Outstanding Leadership in Nursing Education, the Virginia Nurses Association Foundation Leadership Excellence Award for Nursing School Dean, and induction into the Sigma Theta Tau International Researchers Hall of Fame. Dr. Jeffries is a Fellow of the American Academy of Nursing (AAN), the NLN's Academy of Nursing Education, and the Society of Simulation in Healthcare, and an alumna of the Robert Wood Johnson Foundation (RWJF) Executive Nurse Fellows program.

About the Contributors

Cynthia Sherraden Bradley, PhD, RN, CNE, CHSE, earned a BSN from the University of Kansas, an MSN from the University of Central Missouri, and a PhD from Indiana University. She is currently an assistant professor and the director of simulation at the University of Minnesota School of Nursing. She has served as a consultant for simulation programs and has presented at national and international nursing conferences. Her program of research is focused on simulation, debriefing, and preparing faculty for evidence-based teaching and learning methods in nursing education.

Amy Daniels, PhD, RN, CHSE, currently serves as the director of the Debra L. Spunt Clinical Simulation Labs, SSIH Accredited for Teaching and Learning. As an assistant professor, she provides simulation-based education in all clinical programs. Dr. Daniels serves the simulation community in a variety of capacities in both the Society for Simulation in Healthcare and the International Nursing Association for Clinical Simulation and Nursing (INACSL). Dr. Daniels' research focuses on psychological safety in simulation-based nursing education. She teaches nationally and internationally on simulation, debriefing, and psychological safety. Her work is disseminated through presentations as well as peer-reviewed publications.

Carol Fowler Durham, EdD, RN, FAAN, FSSH, ANEF, is professor and director, Interprofessional Education and Practice; director, Education-Innovation-Simulation Learning Environment; and director, QSEN Institute Regional Center at the School of Nursing, the University of North Carolina at Chapel Hill. Dr. Durham has made significant and sustained contributions in interprofessional education (IPE) and is a leader in preparing faculty to integrate quality and safety into their curriculum and their teaching. Dr. Durham is engaged with the Global Network for Simulation in Healthcare (GNSH) to develop strategic integration of simulation to engage teams around stories to improve patient outcomes. She has written for numerous publications and presents internationally, sharing her expertise to enhance health care education. She has received many awards/recognitions for her contribution to health care education and simulation.

Mary K. Fey, PhD, RN, CHSE-A, FAAN, ANEF, is the senior director for teaching and learning at the Center for Medical Simulation; faculty in the Department of Anesthesia, Critical Care & Pain Management at Massachusetts General Hospital; and lecturer at Harvard Medical School. She works with health professions faculty internationally to improve their ability to have reflective learning conversations that hold learners to high standards while still holding them in high regard. She co-authored the publication *Critical Conversations: The NLN Guide for Teaching Thinking* and, most recently, *Critical Conversations: From Monologue to Dialogue*.

Susan Gross Forneris, PhD, RN, CNE, CHSE-A, FAAN, is a former professor of nursing at St. Catherine University, St. Paul, Minnesota, and is currently the director for the

National League for Nursing Division for Innovation in Education Excellence, Washington, DC. She is a member of the 2010 inaugural group of NLN Simulation Leaders and is instrumental in the design and implementation of NLN faculty development resources focused on the pedagogy of teaching and learning. Her research and publications focus on the development and use of reflective teaching strategies to enhance critical thinking. She co-authored the publication *Critical Conversations: The NLN Guide for Teaching Thinking* and, most recently, *Critical Conversations: From Monologue to Dialogue*.

Katie Anne Haerling (Adamson), PhD, RN, CHSE, earned her BSN from the University of Washington Seattle. After serving as a U.S. Navy Nurse Corps Officer, she earned her master of nursing from the University of Washington Bothell and PhD from Washington State University. She is a Robert Wood Johnson Foundation (RWJF) Nurse Faculty Scholar Alumna. Dr. Haerling's primary areas of research include assessing the reliability and validity of instruments used to assess simulation participant performance and comparing learning and performance outcomes between experiential learning activities used in health care education. Dr. Haerling is an associate professor at the University of Washington Tacoma School of Nursing and Healthcare Leadership.

Bette Mariani, PhD, RN, FAAN, ANEF, vice dean for academic affairs and associate professor at Villanova University, is a Fellow in the American Academy of Nursing and NLN Academy of Nursing Education. She was president of the International Nursing Association for Clinical Simulation and Learning (INACSL) and is recognized as a leader for her contributions in simulation and has presented globally on best practices in simulation. Dr. Mariani has spent the last 13+ years dedicated to advancing the science of nursing education and simulation through research and scholarship addressing simulation, educational strategies, assessment evaluation, and instrument development. She has disseminated her work through multiple publications, book chapters, and national and international presentations. Dr. Mariani and her colleagues at Villanova developed unfolding simulations with standardized patients with disabilities for the NLN Advancing Care Excellence Series on Caring for People with Disability.

Patricia K. Ravert, PhD, RN, CNE, FAAN, ANEF, served as faculty at Brigham Young University (BYU) College of Nursing from 1999 to 2020 and retired from her last leadership position as dean (2012–2020). Dr. Ravert previously served as the associate dean – undergraduate studies and the coordinator of the Nursing and Learning Center and Clinical Simulation Laboratory. Before BYU, she was employed as a registered nurse in various roles with Intermountain Healthcare from 1974 to 1999. Her research interests include simulation pedagogy and evaluation of simulation experiences.

Mary Anne Rizzolo, EdD, RN, FAAN, FSSH, ANEF, began her career in simulation in the 1980s, when she designed and developed interactive patient case study simulations using an Apple II and a Sony Betamax video player. She then pioneered the development of interactive videodisc programs that won national and international awards. During her tenure at the National League for Nursing, she was the staff liaison for all the simulation projects: the original research project from 2003 to 2006, the Simulation Innovation Resource Center (SIRC) development project, the Advancing Care Excellence (ACES) unfolding cases, vSim projects, and the project to explore the use of simulation for high-stakes assessment. She has delivered numerous national and international presentations, authored articles and book chapters on the use of technology in nursing, and served on many national and international committees and advisory boards. She currently serves as interim president of the Global Network for Simulation in Healthcare and maintains an active consulting practice.

Beth Rodgers, PhD, RN, FAAN, is Nursing Alumni Endowed Professor at Virginia Commonwealth University, School of Nursing. She has been a professor and has held several leadership roles throughout her academic career, including positions at the University of New Mexico and the University of Wisconsin-Milwaukee. She is known internationally for her work in nursing knowledge, concept and theory development, and has published extensively in this area including two widely used textbooks. She provides frequent consultation regarding theory and scholarly thinking throughout the curriculum, doctoral curricula, and faculty development. In addition to her expertise in theory development, she is well known for her work in qualitative and mixed methods research. She serves on several editorial and grant review boards and has received numerous awards for her teaching, research, and leadership.

Foreword

> Theory not only formulates what we know but also tells us what we want to know, that is, the questions to which an answer is needed.
>
> — Talcott Parsons

The original *NLN Jeffries Simulation Framework*, published in 2005, was well thought out and defined the main concepts needed to conduct high-quality simulations. In the years that followed, simulation became the go-to strategy for nurse educators as the clinical world changed. Clinical sites accepted fewer students, and more experiences became observational, often leaving simulation as the only "hands-on" option available for clinical education.

And then . . . the 2020 worldwide pandemic hit!

Simulation in its many forms, and forms newly created, became the go-to — and often the *only* — teaching/learning methodology available to clinical nursing educators and students worldwide. The concepts of *The NLN Jeffries Simulation Theory* provided a firm foundation for testing new ways of doing familiar things, in settings such as distance and virtual simulation (in its many forms). Initial reports suggest that "learning occurred"; we look forward to seeing those studies in publication.

In this second iteration of the monograph, we see the evolution and maturation of the NLN Jeffries Simulation theory. Jeffries has brought together a team of world-renowned writers and researchers for this edition. This new edition of the monograph provides not only guidelines for using the theory in nursing education, practice, and research but also provides suggestions for future research, just as Parsons suggests.

I'm so looking forward to reading and using *The NLN Jeffries Simulation Theory*, Second Edition, and sharing it with others. I think you'll find it useful, too.

Suzan "Suzie" Kardong-Edgren, PhD, RN, CHSE, FSSH, FAAN, ANEF
Associate Professor, MGH Institute of Health Professions
Boston, Massachusetts
President, International Nursing Association of
Clinical Simulation and Learning

Preface

Nurses have a long history of commitment to theoretical thinking and theory-driven activities. Often, nursing has used theories from other disciplines to describe nursing phenomena, practices, and interventions while dealing with clinical care problems, developing best practices in teaching–learning, and/or demonstrating nursing behaviors. Overall phenomena are described by theories that assist in clarifying relationships with other phenomena so that a nursing action, activity, or strategy can be developed based on the theoretical thinking.

Nursing science depends on theoretical thinking to promote the science and our professional behaviors and endeavors (Meleis, 2012). Through theoretical thinking, organization occurs to assist and support what we know and help to advance and clarify the nature of the disciplines of nursing. The state of the science, whether it is through evidence-based nursing practice or evidence-based teaching, can be enhanced in nursing through the processes nurses use to conceptualize actions founded on theory-based policies and theory-driven practices.

Why are theoretical theory and the National League for Nursing (NLN) Jeffries Simulation theory important? Why is this monograph a crucial contribution to the science of nursing education, particularly in the area of clinical simulation pedagogy? Researchers explore different theories to determine which ones are most useful to build and create knowledge in their field. Researchers desire a theory that can refine and explain the phenomena studied. In practice, clinicians evaluate theories, searching for the best evidence to improve health care and patient outcomes. In education, theories are used to decide what and how to assess in an individual patient; to determine nursing actions; to define the best interventions for patients, families, and communities; and to describe how they all interact. Decisions and the interventions determined can be based on theory or theoretical thinking (a level where there is no organized theory, but which serves as an impetus for theory development).

Having a clear, well-constructed theory around simulations is essential to establish a substantive foundation for research, education, and practice, and to advance knowledge in the area of simulation (Rodgers, 2005). Clinical simulation is a phenomenon defined as a perceived activity or a perceived situation, group of events, and/or situation that replicates real clinical practice. In order to understand a phenomenon, nursing theory is used to identify constructs and explain relationships among the phenomena, to predict consequences, and to provide action from these activities (Meleis, 2012). Nursing theory is an articulation of phenomena and their relationships; in addition, it is a mechanism/strategy to communicate such articulation to the research community and to the research scientists who will use the theory to guide their practices.

The NLN Jeffries Simulation theory is one such exemplar that was developed through theoretical thinking and testing as evidenced by the work done by nurse education researchers (Jeffries, 2016). Contributing to the development of the NLN Jeffries

Simulation theory, several nurse researchers conducted activities exploring relationships of the constructs in the theory to determine and declare the NLN Jeffries Simulation Framework similar to a simulation mid-range theory (Durham et al., 2014; Groom et al., 2014, Hallmark et al., 2014; Jones et al., 2014; O'Donnell et al., 2014; Ravert & McAfooes, 2014). This theory was determined to be a mid-range theory, which is a type of theory that is less abstract than broader (grand) theories, as well as one that addressed certain phenomena or concepts that reflect practice in administration, teaching, or clinical education (Meleis, 2012, Rodgers, 2005). In the past, such works may not have been deemed a theory (Rodgers, 2005); however, contemporary thinking and ideas now discuss theory in words similar to those of Meleis (2012): "An organized, coherent, and systematic articulation of a set of statements related to significant questions in a discipline and communicated as a meaningful whole" (p. 29). This theory, the revised NLN Jeffries Simulation theory, was created through a systematic process that involved robust research and literature review, along with nursing perspectives from those immersed in simulations. This work can be an effective tool or guide to implementation as well as further research. The process of the development of this theory is described in this monograph; with this Second Edition, the literature review and support were updated, providing further evidence of the theoretical constructs and theory determination.

This Second Edition of the monograph provides an updated review of the theory, which explains the phenomenon of simulation. Although there has been no change in the concepts or relationships within this theory, this book presents an updated systematic review of the theoretical constructs and uses of the theory, and highlights future research needs in the area of clinical simulation. Use of the theory in studying the simulation phenomenon does not stop here; the work is dynamic and continues. The challenge to nursing education researchers now and going forward is how to continue to test and use the theory to guide the research in studying the phenomenon to contribute to nursing education science. This mid-range theory provides a way to study the phenomenon of simulation that can facilitate the exploration of best practices, outcomes, and system change through research and development that will contribute further to the discovery of new knowledge and practices.

References

Durham, C. F., Cato, M. L., & Lasater, K. (2014, July). NLN/Jeffries Simulation Framework state of the science project: Participant construct. *Clinical Simulation in Nursing*, *10*(7), 363–372. https://doi.org/10.1016/j.ecns.2014.04.002

Groom, J. A., Henderson, D., & Sittner, B. J. (2014). NLN/Jeffries Simulation Framework state of the science project: Simulation design characteristics. *Clinical Simulation in Nursing*, *10*(7), 337–344. https://doi.org/10.1016/j.ecns.2013.02.004

Hallmark, B. F., Thomas, C. B., & Gantt, L. (2014). The educational practices construct of the NLN/Jeffries Simulation Framework state of the science. *Clinical Simulation in Nursing*, *10*(7), 345–352. http://doi.org/10.1016/j.ecns.2013.04.006

Jeffries, P. R. (2005). A framework for designing, implementing, and evaluating simulations used as teaching strategies in nursing. *Nursing Education Perspectives*, *26*(2), 96–103. doi: 10.1043/1536-5026(2005)026<0096:AFWFDI>2.0.CO;2

Jeffries, P. R. (2016). *The NLN Jeffries Simulation Theory*. Wolters Kluwer.

Jones, A. L., Reese, C. E., & Shelton, D. P. (2014). NLN/Jeffries Simulation Framework state of the science project: The teacher construct. *Clinical Simulation in Nursing, 10*(7), 353–362. https://doi.org/10.1016/j.ecns.2013.10.008

Meleis, A. I. (2012). *Theoretical nursing: Development and progress*. Lippincott Williams & Wilkins.

O'Donnell, J. M., Decker, S., Howard, V., Levett-Jones, T., & Miller, C. W. (2014). NLN/Jeffries Simulation Framework state of the science project: Simulation learning outcomes. *Clinical Simulation in Nursing, 10*(7), 373–382. https://doi.org/10.1016/j.ecns.2014.06.004

Ravert, P., & McAfooes, J. (2014). NLN/Jeffries Simulation Framework: State of the science summary. *Clinical Simulation in Nursing, 10*, 335–336. https://doi.org/10.1016/j.ecns.2013.06.002

Rodgers, B. L. (2005). *Developing nursing knowledge: Philosophical traditions and influences*. Lippincott Williams and Wilkins.

Contents

About the Editor v
About the Contributors vi
Foreword ix
Preface x
List of Figures, Tables, and Boxes xv

CHAPTER 1 **History and Evolution of the NLN Jeffries Simulation Theory 1**
Mary Anne Rizzolo, EdD, RN, FAAN, FSSH, ANEF
Carol Fowler Durham, EdD, RN, FAAN, FSSH, ANEF
Patricia K. Ravert, PhD, RN, CNE, FAAN, ANEF
Pamela R. Jeffries, PhD, RN, FAAN, ANEF

CHAPTER 2 **Systematic Review of the Literature for the NLN Jeffries Simulation Framework: Discussion, Summary, and Research Findings 9**
Katie Anne Haerling, PhD, RN, CHSE
Beth Rodgers, PhD, RN, FAAN

CHAPTER 3 **NLN Jeffries Simulation Theory: Brief Narrative Description 45**
Pamela R. Jeffries, PhD, RN, FAAN, ANEF
Beth Rodgers, PhD, RN, FAAN
Katie Anne Haerling (Adamson), PhD, RN, CHSE

CHAPTER 4 **Guidelines in Using the Theory in Nursing Education, Practice, and Research 51**
Beth Rodgers, PhD, RN, FAAN

CHAPTER 5 **From Vision Statement to Reality: Educational Best Practices Across the Curriculum: EPQ-C 57**
Susan Gross Forneris, PhD, RN, CNE, CHSE-A, FAAN
Bette Mariani, PhD, RN, FAAN, ANEF
Amy Daniels, PhD, RN, CHSE
Cynthia Sherraden Bradley, PhD, RN, CNE, CHSE
Mary K. Fey, PhD, RN, CHSE-A, FAAN, ANEF

CHAPTER 6 **Future Research and Next Steps 65**
Beth Rodgers, PhD, RN, FAAN
Katie Anne Haerling (Adamson), PhD, RN, CHSE
Pamela R. Jeffries, PhD, RN, FAAN, ANEF

List of Figures, Tables, and Boxes

LIST OF FIGURES

Figure 1.1	First Iteration of the NLN Jeffries Simulation Framework	2
Figure 1.2	Second Iteration of the NLN Jeffries Simulation Framework	3
Figure 1.3	Third Iteration of the NLN Jeffries Simulation Framework	3
Figure 1.4	Fourth Iteration of the NLN Jeffries Simulation Framework	5
Figure 3.1	Diagram of NLN Jeffries Simulation Theory	46

LIST OF TABLES

Table 2.1	Evolution of Educational Strategies Variables	20
Table 2.2	Evolution of Design Variables	24
Table 2.3	Evolution of Participant Variables	26
Table 2.4	Evolution of Facilitator Variables	29
Table 2.5	Evolution of Outcome Variables	31
Table 6.1	Themes for Research in Simulation: 2016 Review	66
Table 6.2	Emerging, New Themes for Research Found in the 2021 Systematic Review	66

LIST OF BOXES

Box 5.1	Sample Items from Each Category of the EPQ-C	62

History and Evolution of the NLN Jeffries Simulation Theory

Mary Anne Rizzolo, EdD, RN, FAAN, FSSH, ANEF
Carol Fowler Durham, EdD, RN, FAAN, FSSH, ANEF
Patricia K. Ravert, PhD, RN, CNE, FAAN, ANEF
Pamela R. Jeffries, PhD, RN, FAAN, ANEF

THE BEGINNINGS

In February of 2003, Laerdal Medical Corporation (Laerdal) provided funding to the National League for Nursing (NLN) to support a national, multi-site, multi-method project to develop and test models using simulation to promote student learning in nursing. The NLN issued a nationwide call for a project director and schools that wished to be considered as project sites. Fourteen applications were received for the project director position; Pamela Jeffries was the unanimous choice. There were 175 applications from schools of nursing, and eight project sites were selected.

A kickoff meeting took place on June 23 and 24, 2003, at Laerdal Headquarters in Gatesville, Texas, attended by the project director, all project coordinators, and staff members from the NLN and Laerdal. In preparation for the meeting, everyone was asked to do a literature search and bring any articles that could be of use on the project to the meeting. Since simulation as we know it today was in its infancy in 2003, few articles were found. Even a review of journals targeted to medicine and the military that discussed related topics like role-playing and use of video and CD-ROMs yielded limited useful information. Few articles were research based, and most of them provided only anecdotal data.

Since no theoretical framework for simulation existed at that time, much of the meeting was spent discussing this topic. The project director provided the project coordinators with a review of the literature on constructivist, sociocultural, and learner-centered theories that had the potential to guide the development of a theoretical framework based on a collaborative technology model. Next, small groups worked on exploring various constructs related to the theories and developed questions that could guide the development of instruments to measure the constructs.

Following the June meeting, the project director devoted her time to developing the framework to design, implement, and evaluate the use of simulations in nursing

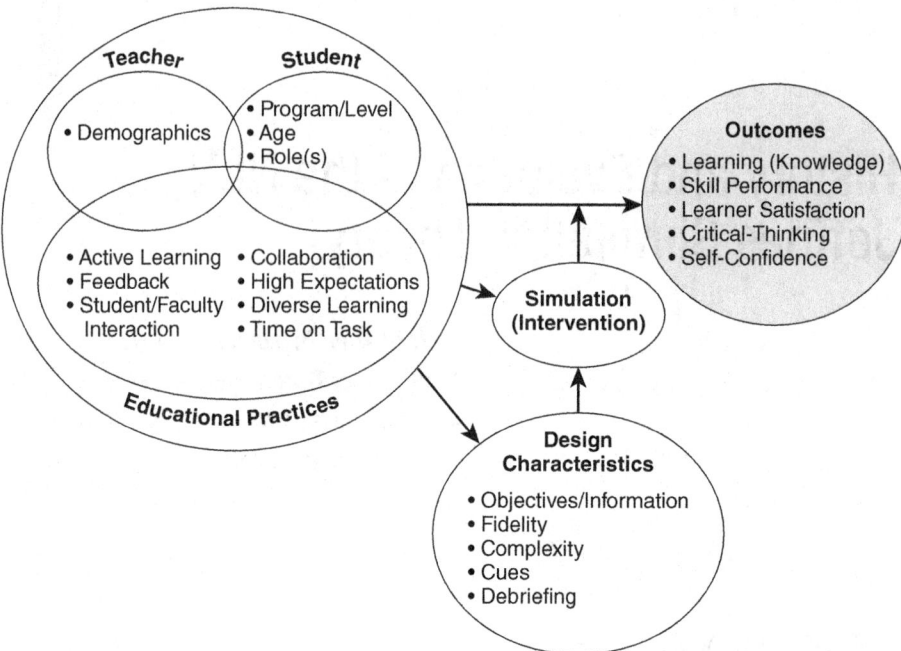

FIGURE 1.1 First Iteration of the NLN Jeffries Simulation Framework. (Reprinted with permission from Jeffries, P. R., & Rizzolo, M. A. [unpublished report, 2006]. *Designing and implementing models for the innovative use of simulation to teach nursing care of ill adults and children: A national, multi-site, multi-method study.*) http://www.nln.org/docs/default-source/professional-development-programs/read-the-nln-laerdal-project-summary-report-pdf.pdf?sfvrsn=0

education. The first image of what was originally called the "Simulation Model" can be seen in Figure 1.1. Jeffries's article (2005) describing the framework and each of its components appeared with a modification of the original model (Figure 1.2); a third variation appeared in Jeffries's book (2007), labeled "The Nursing Education Simulation Framework" (Figure 1.3).

INACSL TEAM EXAMINES STATE OF THE SCIENCE

In the summer of 2011, the International Nursing Association for Clinical Simulation and Learning (INACSL), in consultation with Dr. Pamela Jeffries, convened nursing simulation educators and researchers to examine the state of the science regarding simulation and the application of the Nursing Education Simulation Framework, later known as the NLN Jeffries Simulation Framework. With partial funding from an NLN research grant, the 21 individuals who volunteered for this project were divided into five teams, each assigned to address a different construct of the model: student, teacher, educational practices, simulation design characteristics, and outcomes. Each construct team was asked to examine the literature in light of the following questions:

1. "How is the concept defined in the literature to date?
2. What is the state of the science (what evidence is available) surrounding the assigned framework constructs to date?

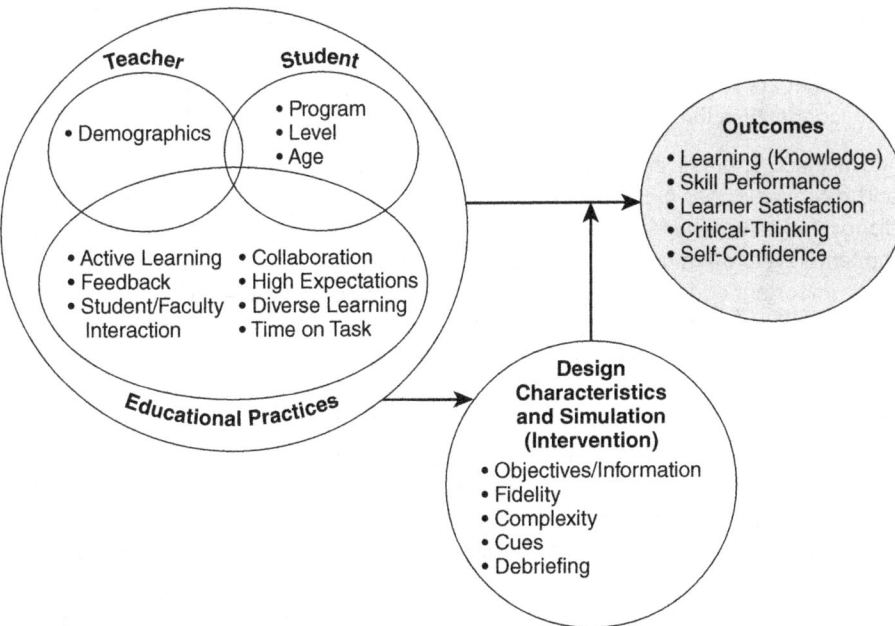

FIGURE 1.2 Second Iteration of the NLN Jeffries Simulation Framework. (Reprinted with permission from Jeffries, P. R. (2005). A framework for designing, implementing, and evaluating simulations used as teaching strategies in nursing. *Nursing Education Perspectives, 26*(2), 96–103.) doi; 10.1043/1536-5026(2005)026<0096:AFWFDI>2.0.CO;2

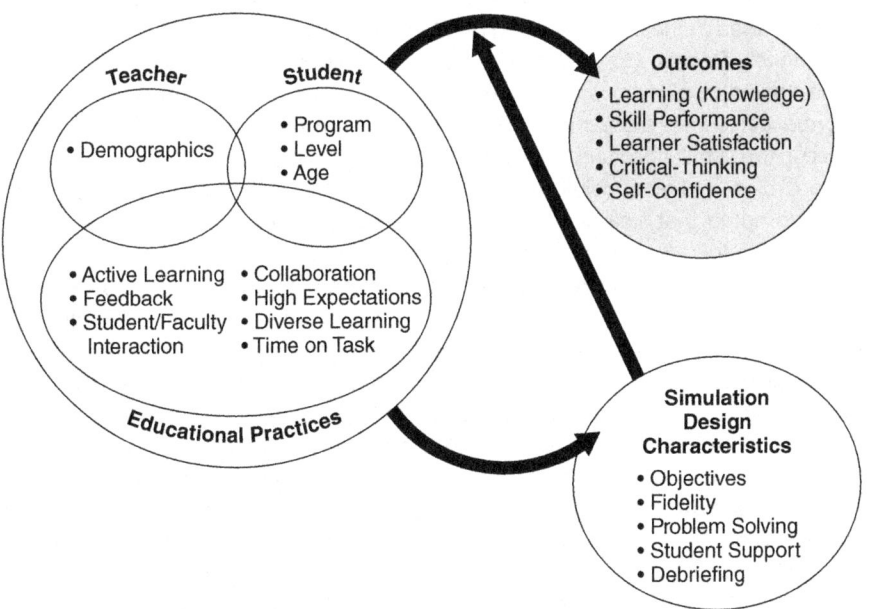

FIGURE 1.3 Third Iteration of the NLN Jeffries Simulation Framework. (Reprinted with permission from Jeffries, P. R. (Ed.). (2007). *Simulation in nursing education: From conceptualization to evaluation.* National League for Nursing, p. 23.)

3. What are the major knowledge gaps and research opportunities in these areas?
4. What are the important future directions for research surrounding the concepts in the framework?" (Ravert & McAfooes, 2014, p. 335)

Hallmark, Thomas, and Gantt (2014) focused on the construct *educational practices,* and discovered that *high expectations* was seldom found in the literature. They also discovered that *debriefing* and *feedback* were different concepts in the literature, but the terms were often used interchangeably. Faculty-student interaction was supported as an important educational practice affecting confidence and retention.

Jones, Reese, and Shelton (2014) discovered that the construct *teacher* was often not defined in the simulation literature. They found that *facilitator* was more consistently used in simulation educational practices and recommended that the term *facilitator* replace the word *teacher.* They noted a lack of reliability and validity for the NLN Jeffries Simulation Framework in the literature.

Durham, Cato, and Lasater (2014) examined the construct *student* and determined that the word *participant* allowed for inclusion of the myriad of roles required in a simulation. Additionally, the review of the literature expanded the list of elements in the original framework from "program, level, and age" to "role/responsibilities, attributes, values, and demographics," providing more comprehensive descriptors of those who participate in simulation.

Groom, Henderson, and Sittner (2014) found that the construct *simulation design characteristics* was "a fundamental guiding foundation for creation, execution, and evaluation of simulation scenarios" (p. 343). They found that the simulation design characteristics — objectives, fidelity, problem solving, student support, and debriefing — were discussed in the literature but did not have strong supporting evidence.

O'Donnell, Decker, Howard, Levett-Jones, and Miller (2014) reviewed the literature for the construct *outcomes* and found that the descriptors *learning* (knowledge), *skill performance, learner satisfaction, critical thinking,* and *self-confidence* were widely discussed in the simulation literature but felt that key outcomes around teamwork, communication, roles, and responsibilities should also be included in outcome measurements. They also noted that "learning outcomes creates a provocative relationship between learner, simulator, educator and environment" (p. 374).

The teams involved in this initial effort to examine the Nursing Education Simulation Framework were plagued by uncertainty about whether they had reached saturation in their search of the literature due to lack of standard terms (Ravert & McAfooes, 2014). Overall, the group found only a few empirical studies and noted variance in the strength of the available evidence to support the constructs. However, the reviews of the literature were instrumental in identifying challenges in the use of the model and uncovered such issues as lack of clarity about the name of the model and how to reference it, as well as inconsistent terminology for the constructs. Two of the research teams identified the need to broaden the names of the constructs from *teacher* to *facilitator* and from *student* to *participant.* These revised construct names were adopted by the NLN and Jeffries for the next iteration of the model (Jeffries, 2012) (Figure 1.4).

Preliminary findings were presented by the team members at the 11th Annual INACSL Conference in June 2012. Manuscripts presenting the evidence for all five constructs

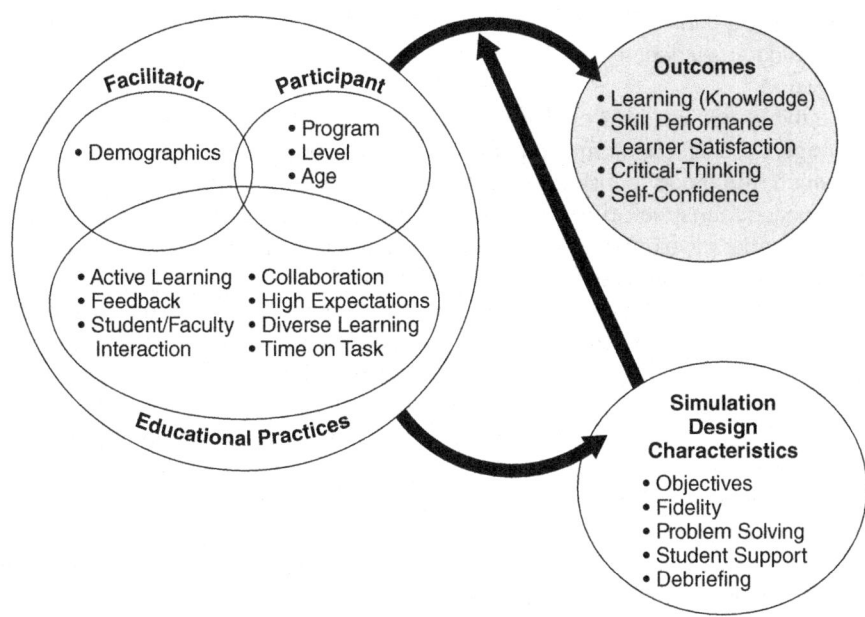

FIGURE 1.4 Fourth Iteration of the NLN Jeffries Simulation Framework. (Reprinted with permission from Jeffries, P. R. (Ed.). (2012). *Simulation in nursing education: From conceptualization to evaluation* (2nd ed.). National League for Nursing, p. 37.)

were published in July 2014 in *Clinical Simulation in Nursing,* providing additional information about the state of simulation, evidence for the constructs, and use of the Nursing Education Simulation Framework. There was consensus across the five research teams regarding the need for further research using the NLN Jeffries Simulation Framework to determine the impact of simulation as a modality for education and research. A published critique of the Framework (LaFond & Vincent, 2013) came to similar conclusions, stating that the Framework offered promise and recommended continued research to empirically support the definitions of concepts and associated variables.

MOVEMENT TOWARD A THEORY

In October of 2012, the NLN received funding from Laerdal to underwrite some of the costs to continue this important work. An internationally known expert in theory development, Beth Rodgers, PhD, RN, FAAN, was recruited to examine the literature reviews provided by the INACSL teams and evaluate the potential for moving the NLN Jeffries Simulation Framework from a framework to a theory. A member of each of the original INACSL teams along with INACSL leaders were invited to participate in this work. Dr. Rodgers held conference calls with team members and requested that they identify significant issues or questions related to the construct that they had previously researched and conduct an initial literature review to determine the availability of research/quality evidence related to those questions. This work was to provide a basis for discussion at a think tank scheduled for June 2013, and to determine the feasibility of constructing an evidence-based foundation for testing and further development of the Framework.

The think tank was held on June 11 and 12, 2013, at the Paris Hotel in Las Vegas. Dr. Rodgers presented information on the theory development process. Over the two-day period, the group focused on identifying goals for the Framework and discussed each concept/construct in the Framework with regard to its clarity, usefulness, and need for further development. The discussion reaffirmed the importance of the Framework and the appropriateness of its components and content.

Dr. Rodgers felt that the NLN Jeffries Simulation Framework could have been called a descriptive theory from the beginning, but recommended that in order to provide a solid theoretical foundation for quality simulation experiences, there is a need to further delineate and clarify each constituent concept or construct in the Framework and to clarify the nature of relationships among the components. This would allow for more testing and can, over time, raise the theory to an explanatory and predictive level. As a next step, she recommended the completion of a comprehensive literature review with high-quality evidence tables focused on completed rigorous research. The intended outcome of such a thorough process would be a comprehensive review of existing research. It would not only clarify the concepts/constructs in the Framework and the relationships among the various components, but would also reveal gaps in the literature and, consequently, clear directions for further research.

In August of 2014, Dr. Katie Adamson was contracted to complete a systematic review of the literature related to the use of the NLN Jeffries Simulation Framework, working closely with and following the guidelines outlined by Dr. Rodgers. The outcomes of Dr. Adamson's work were included in Chapter 2 of the first edition of this monograph. In 2021, Dr. Adamson did a new systematic review exploring the literature from 2014 to date. This new literature review documenting the use of the NLN Jeffries Simulation theory can be found in Chapter 2 of this second edition.

References

Durham, C. F., Cato, M. L., & Lasater, K. (2014, July). NLN/Jeffries Simulation Framework state of the science project: Participant construct. *Clinical Simulation in Nursing*, *10*(7), 363–372. https://doi.org/10.1016/j.ecns.2014.04.002

Groom, J. A., Henderson, D., & Sittner, B. J. (2014, July). NLN/Jeffries Simulation Framework state of the science project: Simulation design characteristics. *Clinical Simulation in Nursing*, *10*(7), 337–344. https://doi.org/10.1016/j.ecns.2013.02.004

Hallmark, B. F., Thomas, C. M., & Gantt, L. (2014, July). The educational practices construct of the NLN/Jeffries Simulation Framework: State of the science. *Clinical Simulation in Nursing*, *10*(7), 345–352. https://doi.org/10.1016/j.ecns.2013.04.006

Jeffries, P. R. (2005). A framework for designing, implementing, and evaluating simulations used as teaching strategies in nursing. *Nursing Education Perspectives*, *26*(2), 96–103. doi: 10.1043/1536-5026(2005)026<0096:AFWFDI>2.0.CO;2

Jeffries, P. R. (Ed.). (2007). *Simulation in nursing education: From conceptualization to evaluation*. National League for Nursing.

Jeffries, P. R. (Ed.). (2012). *Simulation in nursing education: From conceptualization to evaluation* (2nd ed.). National League for Nursing.

Jeffries, P. R., & Rizzolo, M. A. [unpublished report, 2006]. *Designing and implementing models for the innovative use of simulation to teach nursing care of ill adults and children: A national, multi-site, multi-method study*.) http://www.nln.org/docs/default-source/professional-development-programs/read-the-nln-laerdal-project-summary-report-pdf.pdf?sfvrsn=0

Jones, A. L., Reese, C. E., & Shelton, D. P. (2014, July). NLN/Jeffries Simulation Framework state of the science project: The teacher construct. *Clinical Simulation in Nursing*, *10*(7), 353–362. https://doi.org/10.1016/j.ecns.2013.10.008

LaFond, C. M., & Vincent, C. V. H. (2013). A critique of the National League for Nursing/Jeffries Simulation Framework. *Journal of Advanced Nursing*, *69*(2), 465–480. https://doi.org/10.1111/j.1365-2648.2012.06048.x

O'Donnell, J. M., Decker, S., Howard, V., Levett-Jones, T., & Miller, C. W. (2014, July). NLN/Jeffries Simulation Framework state of the science project: Simulation learning outcomes. *Clinical Simulation in Nursing*, *10*(7), 373–382. https://doi.org/10.1016/j.ecns.2014.06.004

Ravert, P., & McAfooes, J. (2014). NLN/Jeffries Simulation Framework: State of the science summary. *Clinical Simulation in Nursing*, *10*, 335–336. https://doi.org/10.1016/j.ecns.2013.06.002

2

Systematic Review of the Literature for the NLN Jeffries Simulation Framework: Discussion, Summary, and Research Findings

Katie Anne Haerling, PhD, RN, CHSE
Beth Rodgers, PhD, RN, FAAN

INTRODUCTION

Systematic review of the literature is a key part of the process of theory development. In the original systematic review of the literature used to develop the National League for Nursing (NLN) Jeffries Simulation theory (2016) the five individual components of the NLN Jeffries Simulation Framework (2012) (facilitator, participant, educational practices, outcomes, and simulation design characteristics) were employed to identify themes, gaps, and key issues that existed in the simulation literature. Findings from the 2016 systematic review helped illuminate what was known about best simulation practices, what research existed to support these practices, and priorities for future research. These findings were used to further refine the framework as it was developed into the current theory. The following chapter describes the original review of the literature and demonstrates how the theory reflects current science and practice in simulation and also serves as an important guide for future implementation and research.

As noted previously, the development and refinement of theory is a vital aspect of the advancement of any discipline. Theory is developed through successive stages and can be accomplished using a variety of procedures. Conceptually focused activities can be used to clarify components; theoretical analysis can determine inconsistencies, gaps, and incongruencies with established theories; and empirical research provides evidence to support the elements and relationships among components of a theory. Theory can be tested directly or, in the early stages of development, existing research can provide guidance as to the order and connections among components. The 2016 review of the literature used this process, focused on the emerging science, to build on the foundation provided by the NLN Jeffries Simulation Framework (Jeffries & Rogers, 2012). The initial framework provided a critical, descriptive view of simulation experiences and essentially represented a theoretical entity of its own. It showed the primary components of the simulation experience, some of the key elements, an order to their appearance in the development and conduct of simulation, and some emerging ideas about relationships and outcomes. The clear documentation of these key elements provided a crucial starting point for the development of the current NLN Jeffries Simulation theory.

A theory is useful to the extent that it provides clear direction both for application and for further research. Over time, in spite of the many contributions that stemmed from the original NLN Jeffries Simulation Framework, it was clear that there was a need to move the work to a higher level. This type of work represented a logical progression in the development of theory in which an original statement of ideas was filled in with more detail. Directions and strengths of relationships emerged, additional pieces were included, and the whole picture presented by the theory became more complete. The progression of theory development can be thought of as a map that, when zoomed out, gives some general shape and major landmarks associated with an area and, on zooming in, makes the details and actual connections among locations become clearer. In other words, more developed theories, or more formal theories, say more about how the person using the theory, whether for practice or research, can get where the person wants to go as well as revealing what will happen if particular routes are followed (or actions taken). While the framework provided some guidance, there was a clear need for a more refined theory, one that would provide guidance along the route of designing and implementing simulation as well as what to do to bring about a desired outcome.

Using the original framework as a starting point, and having identified some of the gaps and needs as well as confirming some of the components in the framework, the existing literature was subjected to a thorough and rigorous review to see what information existed, including both theoretical and research-based evidence, that could be used to refine the theory. This approach was driven by a pragmatic perspective focused on the creation of theory that would provide sufficient guidance to promote the implementation of effective simulation and that also would offer a solid foundation for theory-based research. The development of a theory must be ongoing, and research built on a consistent theoretical foundation will accelerate the process of moving toward theory with relationships among elements and actions that are clear in both direction and magnitude. By continuing both research and implementation related to this theory, it will be possible to determine what constitutes "good" simulation activities and to identify causal relationships along the lines of "if someone does X, then Y is likely to occur."

In some aspects, there was already solid evidence to indicate the preferred practices associated with quality simulation experiences when the original review of the literature was completed. In other aspects, this level of causal relationship was still in an early stage of development. Since the original review of the literature, additional research and the publication of resources such as the International Nursing Association for Clinical Simulation and Learning (INACSL) Standards of Best Practice (INACSL Standards Committee, 2016c) have provided clearer guidance for simulation practice.

The following sections describe the methods and results from the original systematic review of the literature. A comprehensive analysis of the simulation literature was conducted to inform the development of the theory on the basis of thorough consideration of existing research and evidence. This review was guided by the goal of identifying existing research that filled in gaps in understanding regarding simulation, provided needed clarification, and revealed evidence that supported simulation theory. This type of review also revealed gaps or emerging areas of practice that shaped the developing theory. Rigorous and systematic analysis provided an empirical basis for the current version of the theory as well as a rigorous synthesis reflecting the state of the science related to simulation. The procedures described in this monograph also demonstrate the critical interplay of theory and research, with each enhancing and focusing the other in an ongoing process of creating an improved foundation for both practice and research.

For the 2021 publication, updated evidence is included demonstrating progress in simulation science. Examples of additional variables associated with each construct are provided. However, this additional evidence does not represent a full-scale recreation of the original review of the literature. It is important to note also that the more recent findings support the continuing relevance of the theory. The current review strengthens and clarifies the components and the relationships among them. As a result, it provides important updates and insights about the application and relevance of the theory.

METHODS FROM THE 2016 REVIEW OF THE LITERATURE

Garrard's (2014) *Matrix Method for Health Sciences Literature Review* guided the process for the systematic review. This process involved (1) documenting a *Paper Trail* of database searches, (2) constructing *Matrices* for abstracting pertinent content from identified articles, and (3) using the *Matrices* as structured documents for the systematic analysis and synthesis of the literature. The analyses are organized according to the objectives stated by the project supervisor:

1. Discuss the recurring themes, gaps, and key issues.
2. Summarize what currently constitutes best practices and what current research supports.
3. Identify priority areas for which research is needed.

Paper Trail

This review focused on articles from the database Cumulative Index of Nursing and Allied Health Literature (CINAHL) Plus with full text, and the journal *Simulation in Healthcare*. Reference lists from key publications were also used to add depth about specific issues identified in the systematic review. In order to address the purposes of this systematic review, it was important to use the NLN Jeffries Simulation Framework as a guide. However, it was also important to consider literature that might go beyond the boundaries of the existing NLN Jeffries Simulation Framework. Therefore, two separate searches were necessary. The first search was guided by general search terms that corresponded with the five components of the NLN Jeffries Simulation Framework (facilitator, participant, educational practices, outcomes, and simulation design characteristics). The results from this search illuminated literature that was related to each of the components of the NLN Jeffries Simulation Framework but may or may not have specifically referred to the NLN Jeffries Simulation Framework. The second search, specifically using the terms "Framework (in title) AND National League for Nursing OR NLN OR Jeffries OR Simulation" uncovered articles that referred to the NLN Jeffries Simulation Framework.

Paper Trail for Search One

The initial search parameters were "Apply related terms, Research article, Scholarly/peer reviewed journals, and English language." The search dates were January 2000 to September 2014.

Terms: Simulat* in title (to include terms such as simulation, simulator, etc.) AND

Facilitat* OR Instruct* OR Teach* in abstract: 435

Student OR Participant OR Learner in abstract: +559 new references (after deleting duplicates) = 994

Educational practice* OR Pedagog* in abstract: +2 new references (after deleting duplicates) = 996

Result* OR learn* OR skill* in abstract: +853 new references (after deleting duplicates) = 1,849

Objective* OR design OR fidelity OR problem solving OR support OR debrief*: +76 new references (after deleting duplicates) = 1,925 TOTAL

This search was then narrowed using the following major subject headings:

simulations

computer simulation

patient simulation

models, anatomic

education, medical

clinical competence

education, nursing

education, nursing, bacca . . .

teaching methods

internship and residency

students, nursing

education, clinical

students, nursing, baccal . . .

resuscitation, cardiopulm . . .

student attitudes

computer assisted instruc . . .

learning methods

emergency medicine

exercise physiology

outcomes of education

students, medical

education, interdisciplin . . .

virtual reality

emergency care

resuscitation

teamwork

communication

cognition

task performance and anal . . .

user-computer interface

decision making, clinical

emergency service

student performance appra . . .

physicians

disaster planning

educational measurement

emergency medical technic...

heart arrest

multidisciplinary care te . . .

teaching methods, clinica . . .

learning

pediatrics

psychomotor performance

airway management

staff development

This reduced the "hit list" to 1,250 references from CINAHL.

One journal that is not included in CINAHL that provided essential evidence for this systematic review was *Simulation in Healthcare*. Therefore, the same search terms from the CINAHL search described previously were used, yielding the following results. (Note: This electronic journal is only available from 2006 to the present.)

Terms: Simulat* in title (to include terms such as simulation, simulator, etc.) AND Facilitat* OR Instruct* OR Teach* as keywords: 8

Student OR Participant OR Learner as keywords: 19

Educational practice* OR Pedagog* as keywords = 50

Result* OR learn* OR skill* as keywords = 149

Objective* OR design OR fidelity OR problem solving OR support OR debrief* as keywords = 19

Total from *Simulation in Healthcare:* 245

Total from CINAHL and *Simulation in Healthcare:* 1,495 articles and abstracts

Next, systematic reviews within the results list were identified and read (approximately 30) to get an idea of what topics had previously been reviewed. After reviewing the abstracts and titles of the 1,495 articles, and informed by the systematic reviews, each article abstract was appraised for inclusion in the final review based on this question: Is this article essential for understanding "what currently constitutes the best simulation practices?" Using this filter, an initial list of 149 articles was compiled for review.

Paper Trail for Search Two

In order to ensure that existing work related to the NLN Jeffries Simulation Framework was included in the review, additional searches in CINAHL and *Simulation in Healthcare* were conducted using the terms "Framework (in title) AND National League for Nursing OR NLN OR Jeffries OR Simulation." All the filters applied in the first search were used, with the exception that this search did not include "research article" as a search parameter. This, along with subsequent snowball searches using the reference lists of resulting articles, provided an additional 38 articles directly referring to the NLN Jeffries Simulation Framework. The International Nursing Association for Clinical Simulation in Nursing (2011) Task Force on the NLN Jeffries Simulation Framework publications were included in these results. Both conference posters and *Clinical Simulation in Nursing* articles initially were included, but poster presentations that later were developed into articles were eliminated.

These two searches yielded a total of 187 articles. The first was guided by the components of the NLN Jeffries Simulation Framework and the second focused on literature that directly used to the framework. Step two of the *Health Sciences Literature Review* process is described by Garrard (2014): constructing *Matrices* for abstracting pertinent content from identified articles began after acquiring the PDFs of each of these articles (minus 5 percent that were inaccessible). Through this process, the list of articles numbering 153 was reduced even further (115 from the more general "search one" and 38 from the more specific "search two"). In order to limit potential bias for simply confirming the existing NLN Jeffries Simulation Framework, the reviews of these two groups of articles were kept separate for the initial stages of the systematic review.

RESULTS: ANALYSIS AND SYNTHESIS OF FINDINGS FROM THE 2016 REVIEW OF THE LITERATURE

The following narrative uses data extracted from the previously described searches. Initially, two matrices were compiled: (1) the matrix of articles identified using the components of the NLN Jeffries Simulation Framework (search one) and (2) the matrix of articles identified using the terms "NLN Jeffries Simulation Framework" (search two). From these matrices, a list of statements addressing each of the project objectives was compiled. This section addresses the following objectives:

1. Discuss the recurring themes, gaps, and key issues.
2. Summarize what currently constitutes the best practices and what current research supports.
3. Identify priority areas for which research is needed.

Recurring Themes, Gaps, and Key Issues

Three themes from the 2016 review of the literature were "simulation works," "fidelity is important," and "debriefing is where it's at." The following section discusses these original key themes as well as updates to the state of the science for each theme.

Simulation "Works"

A recurring theme from the original review of the literature was that simulation, when compared with other types of instruction, produces positive outcomes. High-quality systematic reviews and meta-analyses clearly demonstrated that simulation, when compared with baseline or no intervention, contributed to improved performance (Cook et al., 2011), and simulation, when compared with more traditional teaching strategies, was associated with superior outcomes (Cook et al., 2013). Evidence in support of simulation was strong and growing and the recently released National Council of State Boards of Nursing (NCSBN) Simulation Study suggested that high-quality simulation could effectively be used to replace up to 50 percent of clinical time (Hayden et al., 2014). While it was generally agreed that simulation "works," the evidence supporting this claim varied in scope and quality.

Satisfaction and Confidence. Evidence from the 2016 review of the literature confirmed that, in general, participants (Rezmer et al., 2011) and educators like simulation. They intuitively believed that simulation leads to improved learning and performance (Baillie & Curzio, 2009; Leigh, 2008). Multiple studies concluded that simulation improved satisfaction and confidence (Kiat et al., 2007; LaFond & Vincent, 2012; Smithburger et al., 2012), and overall, participants enjoyed simulation and requested additional simulation experiences (Partin et al., 2011). Roh and Lim (2014) found that pre-course simulations were the single largest predictor of student satisfaction when compared with pre-course e-learning, observation, and clinical placement skill performance opportunities. Evidence that this fervor may not be universal came from Paskins and Peile (2010), who identified two "camps" in relation to simulation affinity: simulation enthusiasts and simulation non-enthusiasts. Satisfaction and confidence, two items under the "Outcomes" component of the NLN Jeffries Simulation Framework, were widely considered low-level evaluation metrics and there was a need to compare outcomes from simulation with outcomes from other teaching and learning activities.

Comparative Effectiveness of Simulation. Within this original 2016 review, multiple studies demonstrated that simulation produced superior learning outcomes when compared with more traditional lecture or didactic teaching strategies (Cooper et al., 2012; LeFlore et al., 2012; Tiffen et al., 2011). The systematic review and meta-analysis by Cook et al. (2013) confirmed these findings with the conclusion that, compared with other instructional strategies, high-tech simulation produced better learning outcomes. The key issue identified within this theme that "simulation works" was a need for higher-quality research designs and improved measurement practices (Yuan, Williams, & Fang, 2012; Yuan, Williams, Fang, & Ye, 2012) to produce generalizable evidence about the effectiveness of simulation (McGaghie, 2008). One of the primary gaps in this area was the scarcity of valid and reliable instruments for measuring performance (Harder, 2010; Walsh et al., 2012). Further, there was a need to explore additional criteria of "effectiveness" including patient outcomes related to simulation training. Kirkpatrick's (1998) levels of evaluation and translation science (McGaghie et al., 2014) were suggested as model frameworks for measuring the effectiveness of simulation.

2021 Update about "Simulation Works." Since 2016, the literature has shifted beyond the broad question about whether simulation works to more nuanced questions about how specific simulation-based experiences affect learning, behavior, and outcomes; and what aspects or educational practices support learning (Lineberry et al., 2018). Simulation research has come a long way from an overemphasis on satisfaction and self-confidence, but more progress is needed (Cantrell et al., 2017; Doolen et al., 2016). Donohue et al. (2020) demonstrated there was no correlation between self-efficacy and actual clinical skills in a study of simulation focused on simulation and neonatal resuscitation. This further emphasizes the need for higher levels of evidence demonstrating the effectiveness of simulation (in contrast with the over-reliance on measures of satisfaction, confidence, etc.). Examples of studies attempting to measure outcomes beyond satisfaction and self-confidence include de Melo et al. (2021), who looked at patients before and after an *in situ* post-partum hemorrhage simulation, and Craig et al. (2021), who used the Medication Safety Knowledge Assessment (MSKA) to assess knowledge and the Medication Safety Critical Element Checklist (MSCEC) to assess competency after students participated in a structured medication safety simulation. In addition to attempting to evaluate simulation at higher levels, researchers are taking a closer look at how simulation supports (or does not support) important interpersonal abilities such as cultural competence (Lee et al., 2020), cultural humility (Foronda et al., 2018), interprofessional socialization (Rossler et al., 2020), and collaborative behaviors (Cayir et al., 2020).

Fidelity Is Important

The second theme identified through the original 2016 review of the literature was that fidelity is important. The importance of fidelity, generally considered as the degree to which the simulation reflects reality, to the success of simulation activities was underscored by the volume of data around this simulation design characteristic. Comparing levels of fidelity and defining fidelity were the focus of multiple studies.

Comparing "Levels" of Fidelity. At the time of the original review, there was a lack of clarity about the definition of fidelity and, not surprisingly, mixed evidence about whether one level of fidelity (high, medium, or low) was superior to the others. Several studies found similar learning outcomes with various levels of fidelity (Beebe, 2012; Lane & Rollnick, 2007). However, Grady et al. (2008) found higher performance and more positive participant attitudes associated with high (vs. low) fidelity; Butler, Veltre, and Brady (2009) noted that learners perceived that high-fidelity simulation had a greater impact on their problem-solving abilities than low-fidelity simulations. Schwartz et al. (2007) found that human patient simulation had various advantages over case-based learning. Further, when comparing static manikin, high-fidelity simulation, and paper-and-pencil case studies, static manikin and high-fidelity simulation were identified as more effective in offering problem-solving opportunities and feedback (Jeffries & Rizzolo, 2006). High-fidelity simulation was associated with higher participant satisfaction, and paper-and-pencil case study was less effective in promoting self-confidence (Jeffries & Rizzolo, 2006).

In contrast, when doing a similar comparison between paper-and-pencil case study and high-fidelity simulation, Tosterud, Hedelin, and Hall-Lord (2013) found that the paper-and-pencil case study group was more satisfied than the high-fidelity simulation group. Further, Yang, Thompson, and Bland (2012) noted that increased realism in simulation activities was associated with reduced confidence and judgment accuracy among participants. Looking at additional technological capacities such as offering computer-based simulations in three dimensions (3-D), Bai et al. (2012) noted that participants who were exposed to text-based (non-3-D) simulations reported similarly positive attitudes toward simulation as those in the 3-D simulation group. Looking at the fidelity issue through cost-effectiveness lenses, Lapkin and Levett-Jones (2011) found that medium fidelity was more cost-effective, though high fidelity had higher utility.

The "take-home message" from this recurring theme in the research was that it was necessary to identify the appropriate level of fidelity to meet the objectives of specific simulation activities (Blake & Scanlon, 2007). For example, Andreatta et al. (2014) found that an inexpensive fruit model provided adequate fidelity for teaching highly technical operative skills. In another study, the authors confirmed previous findings with their conclusion that transitioning from low to high fidelity resulted in increased confidence (Dancz et al., 2014), confirming findings from Maran and Glavin (2003). In the end, as recommended by Hayden et al. (2014), an "adequate" level of fidelity was necessary as part of high-quality simulation activities in order to ensure high-quality simulation outcomes. The optimal level of fidelity, however, may vary depending on the context and the learning objectives for the simulation experience.

Defining Fidelity. While there was a great deal of literature comparing outcomes from simulation activities conducted at varying levels of fidelity, there was not a consistent, agreed-upon definition of fidelity or what variables should be taken into consideration when determining "levels" of fidelity. Paige and Morin (2013) described multiple dimensions of fidelity including physical, psychological, and conceptual fidelity, each of which exist on a continuum from low to high. Hotchkiss, Biddle, and Fallacaro (2002) used "authenticity" as a measure of realism or fidelity while Dieckmann, Gaba, and Rall (2007) identified multiple dimensions of realism to include physical, semantical, and phenomenal realism. This gap in the literature was addressed by the INACSL Standards of Best Practice: Simulation Standard I: Terminology, in which "Fidelity" was looked at from a holistic point of view including physical, psychological, and social factors in addition to group culture and dynamics (Meakim et al., 2013). A key issue was that simulation researchers had not adopted a single definition of fidelity, which complicated efforts to synthesize and generalize evidence about best practices related to fidelity.

2021 Update about "Fidelity Is important." Since the original publication of this monograph, the INACSL Standards of Best Practice: Simulation: Simulation Glossary (INACSL, 2016e) and Society for Simulation in Healthcare (SSH) Dictionary (Lioce et al., 2020) have provided clarification about the dimensions and complexity of fidelity. The

SSH Dictionary provided definitions not only for high and low fidelity, but for conceptual fidelity, environmental fidelity, functional fidelity, physical fidelity, and psychological fidelity. Similarly, the INACSL Glossary describes the three dimensions of fidelity: conceptual, physical/ environmental, and psychological. These definitions provide useful guidance for researchers seeking to describe and compare the effects of various types and levels of fidelity. The general consensus seems to be that more is not necessarily better and simulationists should aim to utilize the appropriate types and levels of fidelity to support the objectives of the simulation. Examples of ongoing work examining the fidelity include Mills et al. (2016), who used qualitative and quantitative methods to compare how varying levels of environmental fidelity affected participants' cognitive burden and performance, and Harder (2018), who discusses the ethical obligation to support psychological safety and to attend to the psychological and emotional experience of simulation participants, especially highly realistic and emotionally charged simulations.

Debriefing Is Where It's At

Another theme that emerged from the original systematic review of the literature used to develop the NLN Jeffries Simulation theory (2016) was the high value placed on debriefing. Simulation researchers prioritized debriefing as a key component of simulation activities. They recognized its contributions to successful simulation and appropriately focused on several aspects of debriefing, including whether video enhanced or detracted from the simulation debriefing process.

Debriefing Is Essential. Bremner, Aduddell, Bennett, and VanGeest (2006) identified debriefing after each simulation experience as an essential best practice when using simulation with novice nursing students. Hayden et al. (2014) qualified their landmark finding that up to 50 percent of clinical time may be replaced with simulation by denoting that the simulations must be of "high-quality" and accompanied by "theory-based debriefing" (p. 538). Nursing students seemed to agree with the experts and identified debriefing as the most important design feature of simulation (Dobbs et al., 2006).

Clearly, debriefing was and is important, but there have been lingering questions about which characteristics of debriefing were most effective for which desired outcomes. Dieckmann et al. (2009) suggested allowing participants to do most of the talking during debriefing. Bond et al. (2006) found technical debriefing to be slightly better than cognitive debriefing among emergency department medical residents. Cheng, Eppich, Grant, Sherbino, Zendejas, and Cook (2014) found a short debriefing session to be slightly favored over a longer debriefing session. Dieckmann, Molin Friis, Lippert, and Østergaard (2009) explored the interaction between facilitator and participant and found mixed responses about what an "ideal" facilitation/debriefing looked like. These results show that the ideal debriefing scenario may vary among facilitators, learners, and contexts. Variation related to the style or skill of the debriefer cannot be overlooked as a potential explanation for findings related to debriefing scenarios.

Video-Enhanced, Nonvideo-Enhanced Debriefing. One meta-theme within the debriefing theme from the 2016 review of the literature was about the use of video as a supplement to debriefing. Cheng et al. (2014) found negligible differences between video-enhanced and nonvideo-enhanced debriefing. Ha (2014) found that video-assisted debriefing assisted with self-reflection; however, some learners indicated it made them feel "tired" and "humiliated," while other learners said that it boosted their self-confidence. Results from a systematic review by Levett-Jones and Lapkin (2014) about the effectiveness of debriefing affirmed that debriefing was important, but there were no significant differences with or without use of video. While this issue had been extensively investigated, there continues to be reason to question if video-assisted debriefing should be considered the "gold standard?"

2021 Update about "Debriefing Is Where It's At." At the time of the original systematic review of the literature, there was a substantial volume of research on the topic of debriefing. Since then, INACSL Standards of Best Practice: Simulation: Debriefing (INACSL, 2016d) has provided specific criteria to support effective debriefing. In answer to the meta-theme questions about video-assisted debriefing from the 2016 review of the literature, the INACSL Standard on Debriefing notes, "Choose the appropriate feedback technique, which may include face-to-face, numeric, graphical transcripts of performance from equipment, video conferencing or video replay, checklists, scores, and other forms of feedback" (p. S22). In short, video-enhanced debriefing has not emerged as the gold-standard but may be used when appropriate. The newer literature is rich with studies comparing the quality (Ali & Musallam, 2018) and outcomes (Gantt et al., 2018; Wilbanks et al., 2020) associated with various types of debriefing. There is also an emphasis on debriefing after virtual simulations that are sometimes completed asynchronously (Verkuyl, Lapum, et al., 2020; Verkuyl, Richie, et al., 2020).

Best Practices Supported by the Research

While none of the three primary themes that emerged from the 2016 literature review offered definitive direction about what constitutes best practices, there were several beacons of light for those seeking best practices supported by the research. Two of the key documents from this systematic review were previous systematic reviews and meta-analyses about best practices in simulation-based instruction (Cook et al., 2013; Issenberg et al., 2005). Issenberg et al.'s (2005) Best Evidence Medical Education (BEME) review described features and uses of high-fidelity simulations that lead to effective learning. These 10 features were *feedback, repetitive practice, curriculum integration, range of difficulty level, multiple learning strategies, capture clinical variation, controlled environment, individualized learning, defined outcomes or benchmarks*, and *simulator validity* (pp. 21–24). Each of these features also has been supported by other authors and researchers. Cook et al. (2013) confirmed Issenberg et al.'s (2005) features of effective simulation and contributed additional features including *distributed practice, interactivity, mastery learning, longer time in simulation*, and *group instruction*. Of these features, only group instruction was not consistently supported by the literature as a feature of simulation that reliably improved results (p. e851). Thematic analyses of interviews with medical students about their experiences with simulation-based instruction independently (without prompting) confirmed that feedback, curricular integration, repetitive practice, multiple learning strategies, controlled environment, and simulator validity were especially valued by students (Paskins & Peile, 2010).

Educational Practices

Educational Practices were a component of the original NLN Jeffries Simulation Framework that became part of Educational Strategies in the NLN Jeffries Simulation theory. Many of the previously described best practices from the 2016 review of the literature addressed aspects of the educational practices. Table 2.1 describes the evolution of variables associated with Educational Practices from the NLN Jeffries Simulation Framework, variables identified during the 2016 review of the literature, and variables identified during the 2021 monograph revision.

Feedback. The literature examined as part of the 2018 review demonstrated that feedback and expert modeling from facilitators (Abe et al., 2013), as well as feedback from peers (Stegmann et al., 2012), improved participant learning and performance. These multiple sources of feedback and their interaction with educational practices seem to support the overlap in the NLN Jeffries Simulation Framework Venn diagram as well as the arrows indicating the impact that they have on outcomes. Halstead et al. (2011) identified a feedback-rich environment as a theme for describing quality simulation activities. Characteristics of feedback that were supported by the literature included providing immediate feedback about simulation performance (Johannesson et al., 2010) as well as offering participants opportunities to apply what was learned through the provided feedback (Auerbach et al., 2011). Scaringe, Chen, and Ross (2002) found that early in the learning process, both qualitative and quantitative feedback are effective, but quantitative feedback was more effective later in the learning process. Hallmark, Fentress, Thomas, and Gantt (2014) suggested that there was a need to differentiate between feedback and debriefing.

TABLE 2.1

Evolution of Educational Strategies Variables

Variables from the NLN Jeffries Simulation Framework	Variables Identified During Original (2016) Review of the Literature	Variables Identified During Monograph Revision (2021)
Active learning	Interactivity	Pre-brief through debrief
Feedback	Feedback	Feedback
Student/faculty interaction	Learner-centered	Cuing
Collaboration	Interactivity	Theory-based practices
High expectations	Mastery learning, defined outcomes/benchmarks	Curricular integration
Diverse learning	Range of difficulty, multiple learning strategies, capture clinical variation, individualized learning	Diverse learning
Time on task		Repeated exposure
	Repetitive practice, deliberate practice, dose and sequence of activities	

Cuing as a Form of Feedback. Paige and Morin (2013) concluded that there are two types of cues: *conceptual cues* that help the participant achieve the instructional objectives of the simulation and *reality cues* that help the participant navigate or clarify any gaps in the fidelity of the simulation. These investigators suggested that feedback in the form of cuing should be intentional, related to the objectives of the simulation, and practiced prior to the implementation of the simulation (Paige & Morin, 2013). They described how cues may be delivered in a variety of ways. For example, the simulation manikin or other equipment may be programmed to display a response such as an increased heart rate that the simulation participant can palpate on the manikin, or the response may be visualized on the monitor. Similarly, the simulated patient, other role actors, or the facilitator may offer feedback in the form of cues. Binder et al. (2014) found that both verbal and equipment-generated feedback was effective. Garrett, MacPhee, and Jackson (2010) indicated that participants valued timely cues such as patient status changes.

Learner-Centered Practices. The literature included in the original review did not explicitly address student/faculty interaction or collaboration. However, there was evidence suggesting that simulation activities should be learner centered. Nicholson (2012) concluded that simulations should be designed to meet learners' needs, promote learner engagement, and consider environmental safety. Learner/teacher collaboration, such as formative assessment and participant involvement in planning of simulation activities, helped meet participants' specific learning needs (Elfrink et al., 2009). Bremner et al. (2006) and Montan et al. (2014) found that collaboration between facilitators and participants in the planning, implementation, and evaluation of simulation activities was helpful.

Time on Task Reframed as Dose–Response. Numerous studies from the original review of the literature confirmed a dose–response effect with simulation exposure and learning outcomes. Beebe (2012) found that as the number of hours of clinical simulation increased, critical thinking and knowledge scores increased. Both Kennedy, Maldonado, and Cook (2013) and McGaghie, Issenberg, Petrusa, and Scalese (2006) confirmed that longer simulation exposure correlated with improved learning outcomes. Other researchers confirmed that repeated exposure to clinical scenarios through simulation was especially effective (Abe et al., 2013; Auerbach et al., 2011; Johannesson et al., 2010). Finally, while most of the literature supporting repetitive practice and "increased" exposure to simulation did not quantify what an appropriate amount of simulation should be, Childs and Sepples (2006) suggested that a simulation lasting 25 minutes with a 10-minute session for debriefing was too short.

Mastery Learning with Deliberate Practice. A related aspect of educational practices that was supported by the 2016 review of the literature included the use of mastery learning with deliberate practice. In short, mastery learning refers to competency-based educational strategies with standardized outcomes and deliberate practice refers to repetitive rehearsal to develop and maintain knowledge, skill, or ability. Barsuk, McGaghie, Cohen, O'Leary, and Wayne (2009) found that students trained with simulation that included mastery learning and deliberate practice showed improved patient care over students who were trained with traditional methods. Further supporting deliberate practice, McGaghie et al. (2006) found a strong dose–response relationship between the numbers of hours participants spent practicing in simulation and improved learning outcomes. The specific components of mastery learning and deliberate practice cited by McGaghie et al. (2006) included intense, repetitive performance of intended cognitive or psychomotor skills in a focused domain and rigorous skill assessment that provided learners with specific feedback that yields increasingly better skills performance in a controlled setting.

Sequencing. If more is better, it is important to consider how to best sequence elements within simulation activities and how to sequence simulation activities with other learning activities. Evidence from the 2016 review of the literature supported creating each simulation activity with a clear beginning and end (Dieckmann et al., 2007) and sequencing of elements within a simulation to progress from briefing to simulation to debriefing (Cant & Cooper, 2009). Meyer, Connors, Hou, and Gajewski (2011) reported that students who participated in simulation before their actual patient-care experiences demonstrated improved clinical performance. This was confirmed and expanded on by Schlairet and Fenster (2012). These investigators compared different dosing and sequencing schemes for simulation and clinical and found that an "interleaved" scheme, where simulation preceded clinical, was most effective. Further, as previously mentioned, Dancz et al. (2014) found that sequencing simulation experiences so that they transition from lower to higher fidelity increased participant confidence. On a final note about sequencing, it was noted that if simulation is used for assessment, it must first be used for learning (Botezatu et al., 2010).

Additional Educational Practices. Educational practices identified in the 2016 review of the literature that were not covered by the NLN Jeffries Simulation Framework included curricular integration and use of theory. Both of these also were apparent in the review of the literature done for this 2021 update of the monograph.

Curricular Integration. Curricular integration involves the need for simulation scenarios to be standardized and integrated into the curriculum (Cant & Cooper, 2009; Lucisano & Talbot, 2012). This allows for thoughtful sequencing and use of repetition to reinforce concepts (Brim et al., 2010). Further, simulation should not be an add-on to an existing curriculum. It should be thoughtfully used to augment learning and is especially useful for providing experiences that are rare in clinical practice (Cooper et al., 2012). Foster, Sheriff, and Cheney (2008) found that grouping simulation scenarios with other educational activities such as lectures was more effective than simulations alone. Similarly, Deering et al. (2006) used simulation to enforce previous learning, and found that this practice improved participants' comfort with skills.

Use of Theory. Kaakinen and Arwood (2009) found that theory was a missing component in most simulation research, and Rourke, Schmidt, and Garga (2010) agreed that most simulation literature does not adequately address theoretical underpinnings. Wong et al. (2008) suggested that problem-based learning could be used to support an ideal simulation learning environment.

Diverse Learning. Fountain and Alfred (2009) indicated that various components of simulation appealed to diverse learning styles. For example, more social learners benefited from the interactive aspects of simulation while more solitary learners benefited from observation and reflection. Johannesson et al. (2010) found that variation in patient cases enhanced "fun" and the "joy of learning" in simulation.

2021 Update about Educational Practices. The 2021 review of the literature examined the component, Educational Practices, from the earlier version of the NLN Jeffries Simulation Framework and the concept, Simulation Experience, from the NLN Jeffries Simulation theory. Debriefing was still identified as a common topic of research and commentary. While the literature about debriefing was already robust during the 2016 review of the literature, the conversation around the educational strategy of pre-briefing has exploded since the original review of the literature (Dileone et al., 2020; Hardenberg et al., 2020; McDermott, 2020; Tyerman et al., 2019). Other educational strategies that have been developed further since the original review include deliberate practice for mastery learning (Gonzales & Kardong-Edgren, 2017; McGaghie & Harris, 2018; Perretta et al., 2020); the effects of repeated exposure to simulation-based educational activities (Hardenberg et al., 2020); and sequencing of simulation and clinical (Hong & Kang, 2018). Theory also has taken more of a center stage in the simulation literature, both in relationship to deliberate practice for mastery learning (McGaghie & Harris, 2018) and other theories such as cognitive load theory, situated learning, and constructivism (Pusic et al., 2018). Many of the educational practices discussed in the original publication are covered in the INACSL Standards of Best Practice: Simulation Facilitation (INACSL, 2016a) including cuing, feedback, and diverse learning. Several reviews of the literature underscored the importance of curricular integration — a repeat theme from the 2016 review of the literature (Cant & Cooper, 2017; Foronda et al., 2020; Onyura et al., 2016).

Simulation Design Characteristics

Similar to the findings of Groom et al. (2014) and Kardong-Edgren et al. (2008), the 2016 review of the literature largely confirmed the simulation design characteristics construct within the NLN Jeffries Simulation Framework but provided limited substance on best practices. One source of guidance about designing evidence-based scenarios came from Waxman (2010). Drawing from her review of the literature and experience with the Bay Area Simulation Collaborative, Waxman (2010) recommended the use of evidence-based guidelines for simulation scenario development which included: (1) ensuring that the learning objectives are defined; (2) identifying the level of fidelity; (3) defining the level of complexity; (4) using evidence-based references; (5) incorporating instructor prompts and cues; and (6) allowing adequate time for debriefing or guide reflection (Table 2.2).

Objectives

There was overwhelming confirmation in the literature from the 2016 review that simulation activities should be goal directed (Brydges, Mallette, et al., 2012; Dieckmann et al.,

TABLE 2.2
Evolution of Design Variables

Variables from the NLN Jeffries Simulation Framework	Variables Identified During Original (2016) Review of the Literature	Variables Identified During Monograph Revision (2021)
Objectives	Goals and objectives, defined outcomes or benchmarks (multiple)	Outcomes and objectives as "guiding tools" and essential to simulation design (INACSL, 2016e)
Fidelity	Multiple dimensions of realism (Dieckmann et al., 2007)	Clearly describe design features in publications
Problem solving	Multiple dimensions of fidelity (Paige & Morin, 2013)	Examine relationships between design features and outcomes
Student support	Authenticity (Hotchkiss et al., 2002)	
Debriefing	Scenario complexity (Guhde, 2011)	
	Briefing, simulation, debriefing (Cant & Cooper, 2009)	

2007; Garrett et al., 2010; Rosen et al., 2012). Smith and Roehrs (2009) found that clear objectives geared at an appropriately challenging goal were correlated with increased satisfaction and confidence. One of the advantages of simulation is that it effectively allows adult learners to address their self-directed learning goals (Kaakinen & Arwood, 2009). The literature also was clear that learning objectives should guide the selection of simulation modality. For example, Kennedy et al. (2013) showed that virtual simulation offered advantages over other types of simulation because it allowed learners to engage in activities with increasing complexity or difficulty, and provided automated feedback and repetition.

Fidelity

Fidelity emerged as a key theme from the 2016 review of the literature; therefore, it is primarily covered in the Recurring Themes, Gaps, and Key Issues section of this chapter. However, a few aspects of fidelity from the 2016 review of the literature that specifically addressed simulation design are discussed here. Overall, the fidelity of the physical environment was considered an important aspect of simulation design, and appropriate participant orientation to the environment supported success (Cant & Cooper, 2009; DeCarlo et al., 2008; Kiat et al., 2007). Fidelity, as discussed earlier, should be considered a quality beyond the sophistication of the manikin (Howard et al., 2010). Learners may also support the fidelity of simulation activities by wearing appropriate attire, demonstrating professionalism (Hope et al., 2011), and participating appropriately as simulated patients and family members (Nicholson, 2012).

Referring to the design of the simulation, Dancz et al. (2014) confirmed previous findings of Maran and Glavin (2003) with their conclusion that transitioning from low to high fidelity resulted in increased confidence. These transitions should be deliberate and should not take place within a given simulation experience. Deckers (2011) indicated that within a given simulation experience, consistency in fidelity improved learning and that lapses or interruptions within the experience should be avoided. An exemplar for using the appropriate transitions in fidelity for the purposes of specific simulation activities was provided by Matos and Raemer (2013), who used high-fidelity manikins to simulate an adverse event and a standardized patient encounter to practice communication skills associated with error disclosure after the adverse event.

Filming

While most of the literature about filming refers to the simulation design characteristic of debriefing, there was substantial documentation in the literature about the effects of filming and the learner perception of "being watched" as simulation design characteristics. DeCarlo et al. (2008) indicated that being filmed was a barrier to nurses' participation in simulation while Kelly et al. (2014) found that filming ranked low in terms of what "mattered" most in simulation activities. Parker and Myrick (2012) found that observation was considered a "threat" by participants and that disbelief (not "buying in" to the scenario) was used as a defense mechanism to counteract the threat. Acknowledging these potential limitations, Trokan-Mathison (2013) indicated that being watched in simulation had been perceived as less stressful than being watched in clinical.

Table 2.2 describes the variables listed under the simulation design characteristics component of the NLN Jeffries Simulation Framework, variables identified during the 2016 review of the literature, and variables identified during the 2021 monograph revision.

2021 Update about Simulation Design Characteristics. One of the main sources of progress associated with the concept of Design from the NLN Jeffries Simulation theory is the publication of the INACSL Standards of Best Practice: Simulation: Simulation Design (INACSL, 2016d). Similarly, the INACSL Standards of Best Practice: Simulation: Outcomes and Objectives (INACSL, 2016b) provide guidance including the statements "Outcomes are an integral component of instructional and research design," and "Objectives are the guiding tools to facilitate achievement of simulation-based outcomes and the hallmark of sound educational design" (INACSL, 2016b, p. S13). Several commentaries (Cheng et al., 2016; Onyura et al., 2016; Salas, 2016) underscored the importance of thoroughly describing simulation design elements within simulation research publications to help advance the science of simulation. The glaring omission of this detail in the reporting guidelines for health care simulation research (Cheng et al., 2016) was highlighted. Along with the refinement of simulation-based research questions from "Does simulation work?" to "What aspects of simulation support what outcomes?" there is a need for researchers to be more deliberate and explicit about simulation design features in their reporting. For example, a review of the literature by Lapierre et al. (2020) revealed that all studies included in the review resulted in improvement in teamwork, but there were mixed findings related to the retention of these improvements. Clearer descriptions of the design features of the simulation activities would have allowed the authors to uncover what design features correlated with sustained improvements.

Participant

The 2016 review of the literature identified research reflecting the contributions of simulation participants as much more complex than the three variables identified in the NLN Jeffries Simulation Framework (program, level, age). Table 2.3 reflects the original variables from the NLN Jeffries Simulation Framework, the variables identified during the original (2016) review of the literature, and variables identified during the 2021 monograph revision.

Research examined as part of the 2016 review of the literature reflected the documentation of multiple participant-related variables that influence performance including age, gender, readiness to learn, personal goals, preparedness, tolerance for ambiguity, self-confidence, learning style, cognitive load, and level of anxiety (Beischel, 2013; Brydges, Mallette, et al., 2012; Diez et al., 2013; Fenske et al., 2013; Fountain & Alfred, 2009; Fraser et al., 2012; Ironside et al., 2009; Jeffries, 2005; Jeffries & Rogers, 2012; Shinnick et al., 2012). As previously mentioned, various components of the simulation experience appealed to and were effective for individuals with diverse learning preferences (Fountain & Alfred, 2009; Shinnick et al., 2012). Counterintuitively, Beischel (2013) found that a strong hands-on learning style was negatively correlated with learning in simulation. Fraser et al. (2012) found that increased participant cognitive load was associated with poorer learning outcomes. In contrast, learners who set personal goals for simulation activities demonstrated better performance in procedural skills (Brydges, Mallette, et al., 2012). Beischel (2013) found that participants who were more "ready to learn" were less anxious while those who spent more than one hour preparing for simulation activities were more anxious.

TABLE 2.3

Evolution of Participant Variables

Variables from the NLN Jeffries Simulation Framework	Variables Identified During Original (2016) Review of the Literature	Variables Identified During Monograph Revision (2021)
Program Level Age	Age (Fenske et al., 2013) Gender (Diez et al., 2013) Readiness to learn (Beischel, 2013) Personal goals (Brydges, Mallette, et al., 2012; Kaakinen & Arwood, 2009) Preparedness for simulation (Beischel, 2013) Tolerance for ambiguity (Ironside et al., 2009) Self-confidence (Jeffries, 2005; Jeffries & Rogers, 2012) Learning style (Beischel, 2013; Fountain & Alfred, 2009; Shinnick et al., 2012) Cognitive load (Fraser et al., 2012; Parker & Myrick, 2012) Level of anxiety (Beischel, 2013; Leblanc et al., 2012)	Observer role Active participant role (Delisile et al., 2019; Rogers et al., 2020)

Participant Factors Under the Participants' Control

Many participant-associated factors that influenced the simulation experience were influenced by the facilitator, educational practices, and simulation design characteristics, but are largely within the control of the participants themselves. Participants' motivations, enthusiasm, and personal feelings about simulation, as well as their willingness to suspend disbelief, affected their ability to fully immerse themselves in simulation activities (Kiat et al., 2007; Leighton & Scholl, 2009; van Soeren et al., 2011). Further, participants who wore their uniforms and displayed professionalism supported the realism of the simulation experience (Dieckmann et al., 2007; Hope et al., 2011) which, in turn, improved participant engagement (van Soeren et al., 2011).

Participant Factors Under the Facilitator's Control

Some participant-associated factors that influenced the simulation experience were largely within the control of the facilitator. For this reason, they may be considered variables more closely associated with the educational practices or simulation design characteristics components of the NLN Jeffries Simulation Framework. These variables include role assignment, orientation, and group size.

Role Assignment. In relationship to role assignment, Kaplan et al. (2012) found that the role of the observer provided an effective form of simulation learning while Jeffries and Rizzolo (2006) found that role assignment did not affect learning outcomes, but observers rated simulation lower in the area of collaboration. Zulkosky (2012) found that viewing a prerecorded simulation was less effective than participating in a case study and lecture. Kelly et al. (2014) found that students ranked their role assignment in simulation lower than other simulation variables as a contributor to their ability to develop clinical judgment while van Soeren et al. (2011) found that participants valued being able to play the role of their own profession.

Orientation. A Delphi study about quality indicators for simulation demonstrated that participants should be oriented to the simulation environment (Arthur et al., 2013). Bambini, Washburn, and Perkins (2009) found that participants' previous experience with simulation did not affect outcomes for novice nursing students.

Group Size. There is extensive literature about the ideal number of participants in a simulation activity. Clearly, the objectives of the simulation will largely determine the appropriate number of participants, but the following evidence may be used to inform simulation practice. Partin et al. (2011) found that students expressed dissatisfaction when there were more than six students in a group and suggested that the faculty-to-manikin ratio should be one-to-one. Rezmer et al. (2011) found that group size (up to four) had no effect. This would lead one to conclude that best practice might look like four to six participants with one facilitator and one manikin. Some conflicting evidence came from Cook et al. (2013), who found that group training had small negative effects, and Shanks et al. (2013), who found that learning in pairs was more effective than individual learning. Hope et al. (2011) found that small groups were preferred over larger groups.

Participant/Facilitator Interaction. One notable dynamic of the earlier NLN Jeffries Simulation Framework was the interaction between facilitator and participant. The literature clearly acknowledged one area where the two roles overlap. This was in the area of self-directed and peer-led simulation activities. Brydges, Nair, et al. (2012) found that self-directed learning in simulation led to improved skill retention and higher correlations between confidence and competence. In further support of self-directed learning, Boet et al. (2011) found no difference in anesthesia residents' performance when they completed self- or instructor-led debriefing. Similarly, Karnath et al. (2004) found similar learning outcomes with independent or faculty-led computer simulations. In contrast, LeFlore and Anderson (2009) found that instructor-led learning was more effective than self-directed learning in simulation and Marmol et al. (2012) found that tutor-assisted learning was more effective than self-directed learning in simulation.

2021 Update about Participant

Since the 2016 review of the literature, there has been an explosion of research about the value of the observer role. Overall, the evidence demonstrates the observer role is not passive, but rather provides individuals with an opportunity to engage and benefit from simulation in similar ways to more active participants. Delisile and colleagues (2019) conducted a systematic review and meta-analysis including 13 studies to examine the effectiveness of active participation compared with observation. Their analyses revealed no significant differences in reactions (Kirkpatrick level 1) and outcomes (Kirkpatrick level 4) based on role assignment (either observer or active participant), but noted that active participants demonstrated significantly greater learning (Kirkpatrick level 2) than observers. Rogers and colleagues (2020) completed a scoping review and examined differences in learning outcomes including knowledge, clinical judgment, clinical skills, teamwork/collaboration, confidence, critical thinking, and insight/awareness. Their review revealed mixed findings about the various learning outcomes of observers when compared with active participants, but overall supported the use of the observer role in simulation-based experiences.

Facilitator

Like with the participant construct, the 2016 review of the literature revealed the contributions of simulation facilitators were much more complex than the single variable identified in the NLN Jeffries Simulation Framework (demographics). In addition to understanding the theoretical/pedagogical underpinnings of simulation, facilitators were described as needing to be self-aware and to help reduce obstacles that may threaten participants' ability to learn (Parker et al., 2012). Paige (2014) eloquently asserted that nurse educators in this role "facilitate discovery" and emotionally prepare and support students.

Facilitators needed to embrace a learner-centered, "guide on the side" approach to facilitation (van Soeren et al., 2011). Behaviors that promoted this approach included allowing participants to do most of the talking during debriefing (Dieckmann et al., 2009) and recognizing that not all "facilitation" must be led by the "facilitator." Computer-assisted facilitation in the form of voice-advisory manikins was shown to improve hand position and compression rates in cardiopulmonary resuscitation (Diez et al., 2013). Additionally, nonfaculty RNs could assist with facilitation (Foster et al., 2008) and standardized patients (Bokken, Linssen, et al., 2009) and educational/technical support staff are valuable members of the facilitation team (Cant & Cooper, 2009). Further, as discussed previously in the Participant section of this chapter, participants could effectively act as facilitators.

Parsh (2010) interviewed undergraduate nursing students and simulation instructors to identify characteristics that each group thought contributed to effective simulated clinical experiences. Facilitator characteristics that students identified as important included personality, teaching ability, evaluation, nursing competence, interpersonal relationships, and realism. Facilitator characteristics that simulation facilitators identified as important included evaluation, nursing competence, personality, teaching ability, technological skills, designing scenarios, and manipulating equipment. Encouragement and positive feedback from facilitators were shown to motivate participants and improve performance (Abe et al., 2013) while facilitator preparation and training were identified by experts as important characteristics that facilitators bring to the simulation (Arthur et al., 2013). Finally, the INACSL Standard V: Facilitator identified demographics, attributes, roles and responsibilities, and values as important factors describing facilitators (Jones et al., 2014). Table 2.4 describes the original variables from the NLN Jeffries Simulation Framework, the variables identified during the original (2016) review of the literature, and variables identified for this 2021 monograph update.

2021 Update about Facilitator

Since the original review of the literature, the revised INACSL Standards of Best Practice: Simulation: Facilitation (INACSL, 2016a) is the most important development related to the Facilitator within the NLN Jeffries Simulation theory. In addition to confirmation that effective facilitation requires a "high level of educational expertise" (Solli et al.,

TABLE 2.4

Evolution of Facilitator Variables

Variables from the NLN Jeffries Simulation Framework	Variables Identified During Original (2016) Review of the Literature	Variables Identified During Monograph Revision (2021)
Demographics	Personality, nursing competence, interpersonal relationships, technological skills (Parsh, 2010) Attitude (Abe et al., 2013) Attributes, roles, responsibilities, values (Jones et al., 2014) Self-awareness (Parker & Myrick, 2012) Teaching ability (Parker & Myrick, 2012; Parsh, 2010)	Educational expertise (Solli et al., 2020) INACSL Standard: Facilitation (2016a)

2020), there is a growing exploration of different options for facilitating virtual simulations (Verkuyl, Lapum, et al., 2020).

Outcomes

The 2016 review of the literature confirmed the importance of the five variables in the outcomes component of the NLN Jeffries Simulation Framework. However, it made a strong case for expanding the scope to include longer-term educational outcomes as well as the impact indicators from simulation such as patient care outcomes (Brim et al., 2010). At that time, large amounts of evidence existed about how simulation contributed to knowledge acquisition, satisfaction, and clinical skill attainment. O'Donnell et al. (2014) indicated that there was less evidence demonstrating that simulation contributes to self-confidence and self-efficacy, but this finding conflicted with other sources (LaFond & Vincent, 2012; Norman, 2012). A review of the literature by Rosen et al. (2012) found that a larger percentage of articles focused on learner reactions to simulation (31 percent) than on other outcomes such as learning (3 percent), behavior change (21 percent), and outcomes (17 percent).

As indicated at the beginning of this chapter, there was strong evidence at the time of the original review of the literature that simulation "works." In addition to the evidence already provided, the literature demonstrated several novel examples of outcomes from simulation. Yuan, Williams, and Fang (2012) and Yuan, Williams, Fang, and Ye (2012) found mixed contributions of simulation to confidence and competence; simulation clearly improved scores on knowledge and skills assessments but not on objective structed clinical examination (OSCE) performance. Koskinen and colleagues (2008) noted that simulation exercises increase cultural and self-awareness. Simulation performance outcome measures provided valid assessments of empathy (Berg et al., 2011) and assessments of simulation outcomes effectively approximated critical thinking metrics (Fero et al., 2010).

At the time of the original review of the literature, one looming question in the area of outcomes remained: Do gains realized in the simulation environment transfer to the clinical environment to impact patient care? While McGaghie et al. (2014) found that the "downstream" effects of simulation had been demonstrated, Finan et al. (2012) produced evidence suggesting that participants who demonstrated improved performance in the simulated environment did not necessarily perform better during actual patient care. Using Kirkpatrick's (1998) levels of evaluation — reaction, learning, behavior, and results — or translational science terminology, that evidence could be interpreted to mean that, while simulation-based training could and did affect patient care, we could not assume that upstream participant reactions and learning necessarily translated into downstream behaviors and results.

The take-away message from this was that those employing simulation for educational experiences cannot depend on research documenting outcomes such as learning, skill performance in the simulation lab, learner satisfaction, critical thinking, and self-confidence as adequate evidence for the effectiveness of simulation. Like Fisher and King (2013) suggested, there was a need to pursue higher levels of outcome evaluation that would provide information about whether or not learners are ready for

TABLE 2.5
Evolution of Outcome Variables

Variables from the NLN Jeffries Simulation Framework	Variables Identified During Original (2016) Review of the Literature	Variables Identified During Monograph Revision (2021)
Learning (knowledge) Skill performance Learner satisfaction Critical thinking Self-confidence	Self-efficacy (O'Donnell et al., 2014) Behavior change (Rosen et al., 2012) Patient outcomes (McGaghie et al., 2014; Rosen et al., 2012) Cultural and self-awareness (Koskinen et al., 2008) Attitudes and empathy (Berg et al., 2011)	Transfer of learning (Bruce et al., 2019) Patient safety (Harder, 2019; Seaton et al., 2019) Cost-utility (Haerling, 2018) Psychological stress of participants (Judd et al., 2016)

practice. Additionally, there was a need to complete longitudinal research looking at multiple levels of evaluation: reaction, learning, behavior, and results/impact of simulation (Kirkpatrick, 1998).

Recommendations from the 2016 review of the literature regarding effective outcome measurements included triangulating simulation evaluation data with other assessments to assess validity (Mudumbai et al., 2012; Wright et al., 2013). Table 2.5 reflects the original variables from the NLN Jeffries Simulation Framework, variables identified as part of the 2016 review of the literature, and variables identified during the 2021 monograph revision.

2021 Update about Outcomes

Improving the rigor of outcome evaluation continues to be a focus within the literature (Harder, 2019; Prion & Haerling, 2017; Santomauro et al., 2020). There has been tremendous progress since the original review of the literature with additional room for improvement. Seaton et al. (2019) completed a scoping review examining the extent to which simulation improves patient outcomes and identified 15 studies that demonstrated simulation's contribution to improved clinician behavior and patient outcomes (Kirkpatrick's levels 3 and 4). Haerling (2018) examined not only the comparative effectiveness of virtual and manikin-based simulation but conducted a cost-utility analysis to compare the two simulation modalities. The emphasis on translation (Bruce et al., 2019) is another promising sign of progress. Continued momentum in this direction will help answer the "looming question" identified in the 2016 review of the literature, "Do gains realized in the simulation environment transfer to the clinical environment to impact patient care?" Empirical evidence supporting the links between learning and behavior, and behavior and outcomes, will support the logical link between learning and outcomes (Cook et al., 2013).

In conclusion, this narrative has described the methods and results from the 2016 review of the literature including data extracted from two matrices: the matrix of articles identified using the components of the NLN Jeffries Simulation Framework and the matrix of articles identified using the terms, "NLN Jeffries Simulation Framework." These results were used to address the objectives for that work: (1) Discuss the recurring themes, gaps, and key issues; (2) summarize what currently constitutes best practices and what current research supports; and (3) identify priority areas for which research is needed. The findings from this original systematic review of the literature largely supported the components of the NLN Jeffries Simulation Framework and provided insights used to develop the NLN Jeffries Simulation theory. Finally, this narrative has provided updated evidence reflecting progress and insights about the application and relevance of the theory in research and practice. These findings inform the recommendations for future research and next steps in Chapter 6.

References

Abe, Y., Kawahara, C., Yamashina, A., & Tsuboi, R. (2013). Repeated scenario simulation to improve competency in critical care: A new approach for nursing education. *American Journal of Critical Care, 22*(1), 33–40. https://doi.org/10.4037/ajcc2013229

Ali, A. A., & Musallam, E. (2018, March). Debriefing quality evaluation in nursing simulation-based education: An integrative review. *Clinical Simulation in Nursing, 16*, 15–24. https://doi.org/10.1016/j.ecns.2017.09.009

Andreatta, P., Marzano, D., Curran, D., Klotz, J., Gamble, C., & Reynolds, R. (2014). Low-hanging fruit: A clementine as a simulation model for advanced laparoscopy. *Simulation in Healthcare, 9*, 234–240. https://doi.org/10.1097/SIH.0000000000000032

Arthur, C., Levett-Jones, T., & Kable, A. (2013). Quality indicators for the design and implementation of simulation experiences: A Delphi study. *Nurse Education Today, 33*(11), 1357–1361. https://doi.org/10.1016/j.nedt.2012.07.012

Auerbach, M., Kessler, D., & Foltin, J. C. (2011). Repetitive pediatric simulation resuscitation training. *Pediatric Emergency Care, 27*(1), 29–31. https://doi.org/10.1097/PEC.0b013e3182043f3b

Bai, X., Duncan, R. O., Horowitz, B. P., Graffeo, J. M., Glodstein, S. L., & Lavin, J. (2012). The added value of 3D simulations in healthcare education. *International Journal of Nursing Education, 4*(2), 67–72. Retrieved from http://search.ebscohost.com/login.aspx?direct=true&db=rzh&AN=2011793111&site=ehost-live

Baillie, L., & Curzio, J. (2009). Students' and facilitators' perceptions of simulation in practice learning. *Nurse Education in Practice, 9*(5), 297–306. https://doi.org/10.1016/j.nepr.2008.08.007

Bambini, D., Washburn, J., & Perkins, R. (2009). Outcomes of clinical simulation for novice nursing students: Communication, confidence, clinical judgment. *Nursing Education Perspectives, 30*(2), 79–82. https://go-gale-com.offcampus.lib.washington.edu/ps/i.do?p=AONE&u=wash_main&id=GALE%7CA198994353&v=2.1&it=r

Barsuk, J. H., McGaghie, W. C., Cohen, E. R., O'Leary, K., & Wayne, D. B. (2009). Simulation-based mastery learning reduces complications during central venous catheter insertion in a medical intensive care unit. *Critical Care Medicine, 37*(10), 2697–2701. Retrieved from http://search.ebscohost.com/login.aspx?direct=true&db=rzh&AN=2010459626&site=ehostlive

Beebe, R. I. (2012). *Relationship between fidelity and dose of human patient simulation, critical thinking skills, and knowledge in an associate degree nursing program*. West Virginia University. Doctoral dissertation. Retrieved from UMI number 3538233.

Beischel, K. P. (2013). Variables affecting learning in a simulation experience: A mixed methods study. *Western Journal of Nursing Research, 35*(2), 226–247.

Berg, K., Majdan, J. F., Berg, D., Veloski, J., & Hojat, M. (2011). A comparison of medical students' self-reported empathy with simulated patients' assessments of the students' empathy. *Medical Teacher, 33*(5), 388–391. https://doi.org/10.3109/0142159X.2010.530319

Binder, C., Schmölzer, G. M., O'Reilly, M., Schwaberger, B., Urlesberger, B., & Pichler, G. (2014). Human or monitor feedback to improve mask ventilation during simulated neonatal cardiopulmonary resuscitation. *Archives of Disease in Childhood — Fetal & Neonatal Edition, 99*(2), F120–123. https://doi.org/10.1136/archdischild-2013-304311

Blake, C., & Scanlon, E. (2007). Reconsidering simulations in science education at a distance: Features of effective use. *Journal of Computer Assisted Learning, 23*(6), 491–502. https://doi.org/10.1111/j.1365-2729.2007.00239.x

Boet, S., Bould, M. D., Bruppacher, H. R., Desjardins, F., Chandra, D. B., & Naik, V. N. (2011). Looking in the mirror: Self-debriefing versus instructor debriefing for simulated crises. *Critical Care Medicine, 39*(6), 1377–1381. https://doi.org/10.1097/CCM.0b013e31820eb8be

Bokken, L., Linssen, T., Scherpbier, A., van der Vleuten, C., & Rethans, J. (2009). Feedback by simulated patients in undergraduate medical education: A systematic review of the literature. *Medical Education, 43*(3), 202–210. https://doi.org/10.1111/j.1365-2923.2008.03268.x

Bokken, L., Van Dalen, J., Scherpbier, A., van der Vleuten, C., & Rethans, J. (2009). Lessons learned from an adolescent simulated patient educational program: Five years of experience. *Medical Teacher, 31*(7), 605–612. https://doi.org/10.1080/01421590802208891

Bond, W. F., Deitrick, L. M., Eberhardt, M., Barr, G. C., Kane, B. G., Worrilow, C. C.,

Arnold, D. C., & Croskerry, P. (2006). Cognitive versus technical debriefing after simulation training. *Academic Emergency Medicine, 13*(3), 276–283. Retrieved from http://search.ebscohost.com/login.aspx?direct=true&db=rzh&AN=2009231674&site=ehost-live

Botezatu, M., Hult, H., Tessma, M. K., & Fors, U. (2010). Virtual patient simulation for learning and assessment: Superior results in comparison with regular course exams. *Medical Teacher, 32*(10), 845–850. https://doi.org/10.3109/01421591003695287

Bremner, M. N., Aduddell, K., Bennett, D. N., & VanGeest, J. B. (2006). The use of human patient simulators: Best practices with novice nursing students. *Nurse Educator, 31*(4), 170–174. Retrieved from http://search.ebscohost.com/login.aspx?direct=true&db=rzh&AN=2009251311&site=ehost-live

Brim, N., Venkatan, S., Gordon, J., & Alexander, E. (2010). Long-term educational impact of a simulator curriculum on medical student education in an internal medicine clerkship. *Simulation in Healthcare, 5,* 75–81. https://doi.org/10.1097/SIH.0b013e3181ca8edc

Bruce, R., Levett-Jones, T., & Courtney-Pratt, H. (2019, October). Transfer of learning from university-based simulation experiences to nursing students' future clinical practice: An exploratory study. *Clinical Simulation in Nursing, 35*(C), 17–24. https://doi.org/10.1016/j.ecns.2019.06.003

Brydges, R., Mallette, C., Pollex, H., Carnahan, H., & Dubrowski, A. (2012). Evaluating the influence of goal setting on intravenous catheterization skill acquisition and transfer in a hybrid simulation training context. *Simulation in Healthcare, 7,* 236–242. https://doi.org/10.1097/SIH.0b013e31825993f2

Brydges, R., Nair, P., Ma, I., Shanks, D., & Hatala, R. (2012). Directed self-regulated learning versus instructor-regulated learning in simulation training. *Medical Education, 46*(7), 648–656. https://doi.org/10.1111/j.1365-2923.2012.04268.x

Butler, K. W., Veltre, D. E., & Brady, D. S. (2009). Implementation of active learning pedagogy comparing low-fidelity simulation versus high-fidelity simulation in pediatric nursing education. *Clinical Simulation in Nursing, 5*, e129–e136. https://doi.org/10.1016/j.ecns.2009.03.118

Cant, R. P., & Cooper, S. J. (2009). Simulation-based learning in nurse education: Systematic review. *Journal of Advanced Nursing, 66*(1), 3–15. https://doi.org/10.1111/j.1365-2648.2009.05240.x

Cant, R. P., & Cooper, S. J. (2017). Use of simulation-based learning in undergraduate nurse education: An umbrella systematic review. *Nurse Education Today, 49*, 63–71. doi: 10.1016/j.nedt.2016.11.015

Cantrell, M. A., Franklin, A., Leighton, K., & Carlson, A. (2017, December). The evidence in simulation-based learning experiences in nursing education and practice: An umbrella review. *Clinical Simulation in Nursing, 13*(12), 634–667. https://doi.org/10.1016/j.ecns.2017.08.004

Cayir, E., Owen, J. A., Brashers, T., Haizlip, J., & Cunningham, T. (2020). Measuring compassionate care among interprofessional health care teams: Developing and testing the feasibility of a collaborative behaviors observational assessment tool. *Clinical Simulation in Nursing, 49*, 1–8. https://doi.org/10.1016/j.ecns.2020.03.011

Cheng, A., Eppich, W., Grant, V., Sherbino, J., Zendejas, B., & Cook, D. A. (2014). Debriefing for technology-enhanced simulation: A systematic review and meta-analysis. *Medical Education, 48*(7), 657–666. https://doi.org/10.1111/medu.12432

Cheng, A., Kessler, D., Mackinnon, R., Chang, T. P., Nadkarni, V. M., Hunt, E. A., Duval-Arnould, J., Lin, Y., Cook, D. A., Pusic, M., Hui, J., Moher, D., Egger, M., Auerbach, M., & International Network for Simulation-based Pediatric Innovation, Research, and Education (INSPIRE) Reporting Guidelines Investigators. (2016). Reporting guidelines for health care simulation research: Extensions to the CONSORT and STROBE statements. *Simulation in Healthcare, 11*(4), 238–248. https://doi.org/10.1097/SIH.0000000000000150

Cheng, A., Nadkarni, V. M., Chang, T., & Auerbach, M. (2016). Highlighting instructional design features in reporting guidelines for health care simulation research. *Simulation in Healthcare, 11*(5), 363–364. doi: 10.1097/SIH.0000000000000202

Childs, J. C., & Sepples, S. (2006). Clinical teaching by simulation: Lessons learned from a complex patient care scenario. *Nursing Education Perspectives, 27*(3), 154–158. https://link.gale.com/apps/doc/A147109028/AONE?u=wash_main&sid=bookmark-AONE&xid=14ed0d77

Cook, D. A., Hamstra, S. J., Brydges, R., Zendejas, B., Szostek, J. H., Wang, A. T., Erwin, P. J., & Hatala, R. (2013). Comparative effectiveness of instructional design features in simulation-based education: Systematic review and meta-analysis. *Medical Teacher, 35*(1), e844–875. https://doi.org/10.3109/0142159X.2012.714886

Cook, D. A., Hatala, R., Brydges, R., Zendejas, B., Szostek, J. H., Wang, A. T., Erwin, P. J., & Hamstra, S. J. (2011). Technology-enhanced simulation for health professions education: A systematic review and meta-analysis. *JAMA: The Journal of the American Medical Association, 306*(9), 978–988. https://doi.org/10.1001/jama.2011.1234

Cooper, S., Cant, R., Porter, J., Bogossian, F., McKenna, L., Brady, S., & Fox-Young, S. (2012). Simulation based learning in midwifery education: A systematic review. *Women & Birth, 25*(2), 64–78. https://doi.org/10.1016/j.wombi.2011.03.004

Craig, S. J., Kastello, J. C., Cieslowski, B. J., & Rovnyak, V. (2021). Simulation strategies to increase nursing student clinical competence in safe medication administration practices: A quasi-experimental study. *Nurse Education Today, 96*, 104605. https://doi.org/10.1016/j.nedt.2020.104605

Dancz, C., Sun, V., Moon, H., Chen, J., & Ozel, B. (2014). Comparison of 2 simulation models for teaching obstetric anal sphincter repair. *Simulation in Healthcare, 9*, 325–330. https://doi.org/10.1097/SIH.0000000000000043

de Melo, B. C. P., Van der Vleuten, C. P. M., Muijtjens, A. M. M., Rodrigues Falbo, A., Katz, L., & Van Merriënboer, J. J. G. (2021). Effects of an instructional design based postpartum hemorrhage simulation training on patient outcomes: An uncontrolled before-and-after study. *Journal of Maternal-Fetal & Neonatal Medicine, 34*(2), 245–252. https://doi-org.offcampus.lib.washington.edu/10.1080/14767058.2019.1606195

DeCarlo, D., Collingridge, D., Grant, C., & Ventre, K. (2008). Factors influencing nurses' attitudes toward simulation-based education. *Simulation in Healthcare, 3,* 90–96. https://doi.org/10.1097/SIH.0b013e318165819e

Deckers, C. (2011). *Designing high fidelity simulation to maximize student registered nursing decision-making ability*. Pepperdine University. Doctoral dissertation. Retrieved from UMI Number 3449818.

Deering, S., Hodor, J., Wylen, M., Poggi, S., Nielsen, P., & Satin, A. (2006). Additional training with an obstetric simulator improves medical student comfort with basic procedures. *Simulation in Healthcare, 1*(1), 32–34. Retrieved from http://ovidsp.ovid.com/ovidweb.cgi?T=JS&PAGE=reference&D=ovfth&NEWS=N&AN=01266021-200600110-00003

Delisle, M., Ward, M., Pradarelli, J., Panda, N., Howard, J., & Hannenberg, A. (2019). Comparing the learning effectiveness of healthcare simulation in the observer versus active role: Systematic review and meta-analysis. *Simulation in Healthcare, 14*(5), 318–332. doi: 10.1097/SIH.0000000000000377

Dieckmann, P., Gaba, D., & Rall, M. (2007). Deepening the theoretical foundations of patient simulation as social practice. *Simulation in Healthcare, 2,* 183–193. https://doi.org/10.1097/SIH.0b013e3180f637f5

Dieckmann, P., Molin Friis, S., Lippert, A., & Østergaard, D. (2009). The art and science of debriefing in simulation: Ideal and practice. *Medical Teacher, 31*(7), e287–e294. Retrieved from http://search.ebscohost.com/login.aspx?direct=true&db=rzh&AN=2010396241&site=ehost-live

Diez, N., Rodriguez-Diez, M., Nagore, D., Fernandez, S., Ferrer, M., & Beunza, J. (2013). A randomized trial of cardiopulmonary resuscitation training for medical students: Voice advisory mannequin compared to guidance provided by an instructor. *Simulation in Healthcare, 8,* 234–241. https://doi.org/10.1097/SIH.0b013e31828e7196

Dileone, C., Chyun, D., Diaz, D., & Maruca, A. (2020). An examination of simulation prebriefing in nursing education. *Nursing Education Perspectives, 41*(6), 345–348. doi: 10.1097/01.NEP.0000000000000689

Dobbs, C., Sweitzer, V., & Jeffries, P. (2006). Testing simulation design features using an insulin management simulation in nursing education. *Clinical Simulation in Nursing, 2*(1), e17–e22. https://doi.org/10.1016/j.ecns.2009.05.012

Donohue, L. T., Underwood, M. A., & Hoffman, K. R. (2020). Relationship between self-efficacy and performance of simulated neonatal chest compressions and ventilation. *Simulation in Healthcare, 15*(6), 377–381. doi: 10.1097/SIH.0000000000000446

Doolen, J., Mariani, B., Atz, T., Horsley, T. L., Rourke, J. O', McAfee, K., & Cross, C. L. (2016, June). High-fidelity simulation in undergraduate nursing education: A review of simulation reviews. *Clinical Simulation in Nursing, 12*(7), 290–302. http://doi.org/10.1016/j.ecns.2016.01.009

Elfrink, V. L., Nininger, J., Rohig, L., & Lee, J. (2009). The case for group planning in human patient simulation. *Nursing Education Perspectives, 30*(2), 83–86.

Fenske, C. L., Harris, M. A., Aebersold, M. L., & Hartman, L. S. (2013). Perception versus reality: A comparative study of the clinical judgment skills of nurses during a simulated activity. *Journal of Continuing Education in Nursing, 44*(9), 399–405. https://doi.org/10.3928/00220124-20130701-67

Fero, L. J., O'Donnell, J., Zullo, T. G., Dabbs, A. V., Kitutu, J., Samosky, J. T., & Hoffman, L. A. (2010). Critical thinking skills in nursing students: Comparison of simulation-based performance with metrics. *Journal of Advanced Nursing, 66*(10), 2182–2193. https://doi.org/10.1111/j.1365-2648.2010.05385.x

Finan, E., Bismilla, Z., Campbell, C., LeBlanc, V., Jefferies, A., & Whyte, H. E. (2012). Improved procedural performance following a simulation training session may not be transferable to the clinical environment. *Journal of Perinatology, 32*(7), 539–544. https://doi.org/10.1038/jp.2011.141

Fisher, D., & King, L. (2013). An integrative literature review on preparing nursing students through simulation to recognize and respond to the deteriorating patient. *Journal of Advanced Nursing, 69*(11), 2375–2388. https://doi.org/10.1111/jan.12174

Foronda, C. L., Baptiste, D.-L., Pfaff, T., Velez, R., Reinholdt, M., Sanchez, M., & Hudson, K. W. (2018, February). Cultural competency and cultural humility in simulation-based education: An integrative review. *Clinical Simulation in Nursing, 15*, 42–60. https://doi.org/10.1016/j.ecns.2017.09.006

Foronda, C. L., Fernandez-Burgos, M., Nadeau, C., Kelley, C. N., & Henry, M. N. (2020). Virtual simulation in nursing education: A systematic review spanning 1996 to 2018. *Simulation in Healthcare, 15*(1), 46–54. doi: 10.1097/SIH.0000000000000411

Foster, J. G., Sheriff, S., & Cheney, S. (2008). Using nonfaculty registered nurses to facilitate high-fidelity human patient simulation activities. *Nurse Educator, 33*(3), 137–141. Retrieved from http://search.ebscohost.com/login.aspx?direct=true&db=rzh&AN=2009932986&site=ehost-live

Fountain, R. A., & Alfred, D. (2009). Student satisfaction with high-fidelity simulation: Does it correlate with learning styles? *Nursing Education Perspectives, 30*(2), 96–98. Retrieved from http://search.ebscohost.com/login.aspx?direct=true&db=rzh&AN=2010258647&site=ehost-live

Fraser, K., Ma, I., Teteris, E., Baxter, H., Wright, B., & McLaughlin, K. (2012). Emotion, cognitive load and learning outcomes during simulation training. *Medical Education, 46*(11), 1055–1062. https://doi.org/10.1111/j.1365-2923.2012.04355.x

Gantt, L. T., Overton, S. H., Avery, J., Swanson, M., & Elhammoumi, C. V. (2018, April). Comparison of debriefing methods and learning outcomes in human patient simulation. *Clinical Simulation in Nursing, 17*, 7–13. https://doi.org/10.1016/j.ecns.2017.11.012

Garrard, J. (2014). Health sciences literature review made easy. In *The matrix method* (4th ed.). Jones & Bartlett Learning.

Garrett, B., MacPhee, M., & Jackson, C. (2010). High-fidelity patient simulation: Considerations for effective learning. *Nursing Education Perspectives, 31*(5), 309–313. PMID: 21086870.

Gonzalez, L., & Kardong-Edgren, S. (2017, January). Deliberate practice for mastery learning in nursing. *Clinical Simulation in Nursing, 13*(1), 10–14. https://doi.org/10.1016/j.ecns.2016.10.005

Grady, J. L., Kehrer, R. G., Trusty, C. E., Entin, E. B., Entin, E. E., & Brunye, T. T. (2008). Learning nursing procedures: The influence of simulator fidelity and student gender on teaching effectiveness. *Journal of Nursing Education, 47*(9), 403–408. https://doi.org/10.3928/01484834-20080901-09

Groom, J. A., Henderson, D., & Sittner, B. J. (2014). NLN/Jeffries Simulation Framework state of the science project: Simulation design characteristics. *Clinical Simulation in Nursing, 10*(7), 337–344. https://doi.org/10.1016/j.ecns.2013.02.004

Guhde, J. (2011). Nursing students' perceptions of the effect on critical thinking, assessment, and learner satisfaction in simple versus complex high-fidelity simulation scenarios. *Journal of Nursing Education, 50*(2), 73–78. https://doi.org/10.3928/01484834-20101130-03

Ha, E. (2014). Attitudes toward video-assisted debriefing after simulation in undergraduate nursing students: An application of Q methodology. *Nurse Education Today, 34*(6), 978–984. https://doi.org/10.1016/j.nedt.2014.01.003

Haerling, K. A. (2018). Cost-utility analysis of virtual and mannequin-based simulation. *Simulation in Healthcare, 13*(1), 1–40. doi: 10.1097/SIH.0000000000000280

Hallmark, B., Fentress, B. F., Thomas, C. M., & Gantt, L. (2014). The educational practices construct of the NLN/Jeffries Simulation Framework: State of the science. *Clinical Simulation in Nursing, 10*(7), 345–352. https://doi.org/10.1016/j.ecns.2013.04.006

Halstead, J. A., Phillips, J. M., Koller, A., Hardin, K., Porter, M. L., & Dwyer, J. S. (2011). Preparing nurse educators to use simulation technology: A consortium model for practice and education. *Journal of Continuing Education in Nursing, 42*(11), 496–502. https://doi.org/10.3928/00220124-20110502-01

Hardenberg, J., Rana, I., & Tori, K. (2020, November). Evaluating impact of repeated exposure to high fidelity simulation: Skills acquisition and stress levels in postgraduate critical care nursing students. *Clinical Simulation in Nursing, 48*(C), 96–102. https://doi.org/10.1016/j.ecns.2020.06.002

Harder, B. N. (2010). Use of simulation in teaching and learning in health sciences: A systematic review. *Journal of Nursing Education, 49*(1), 23–28. https://doi.org/10.3928/01484834-20090828-08

Harder, N. (2018). Dealing with the fidelity of simulation-based learning. *Clinical Simulation in Nursing, 25*, 20–21. https://doi.org/10.1016/j.ecns.2018.10.004

Harder, N. (2019). Simulation and patient safety: Continuing to provide evidence. *Clinical Simulation in Nursing, 29*, 38–39. https://doi.org/10.1016/j.ecns.2019.03.006

Hayden, J. K., Smiley, R. A., Alexander, M., Kardong-Edgren, S., & Jeffries, P. R. (2014). The NCSBN National Simulation Study: A longitudinal, randomized, controlled study replacing clinical hours with simulation in prelicensure nursing education. *Journal of Nursing Regulation, 5*(2S), S1–S63. https://doi.org/10.1016/S2155-8256(15)30062-4

Hope, A., Garside, J., & Prescott, S. (2011). Rethinking theory and practice: Pre-registration student nurses experiences of simulation teaching and learning in the acquisition of clinical skills in preparation for practice. *Nurse Education Today, 31*(7), 711–715. https://doi.org/10.1016/j.nedt.2010.12.011

Hotchkiss, M. A., Biddle, C., & Fallacaro, M. (2002). Assessing the authenticity of the human simulation experience in anesthesiology. *AANA Journal, 70*(6), 470–473. Retrieved from http://search.ebscohost.com/login.aspx?direct=true&db=rzh&AN=2003035287&site=ehost-live

Howard, V. M., Ross, C., Mitchell, A. M., & Nelson, G. M. (2010). Human patient simulators and interactive case studies: A comparative analysis of learning outcomes and student perceptions. *CIN: Computers, Informatics, Nursing, 28*(1), 42–48. https://doi.org/10.1097/NCN.0b013e3181c04939

INACSL Standards Committee. (2016a, December). INACSL Standards of Best Practice: Simulation: Facilitation. *Clinical Simulation in Nursing, 12*, S16–S20. https://doi.org/10.1016/j.ecns.2016.09.007

INACSL Standards Committee. (2016b, December). INACSL Standards of Best Practice: Simulation: Outcomes and objectives. *Clinical Simulation in Nursing, 12*, S13–S15. https://doi.org/10.1016/j.ecns.2016.09.006

INACSL Standards Committee. (2016c, December). INACSL Standards of Best Practice: Simulation: Simulation. *Clinical Simulation in Nursing, 12*, S5–S50. https://doi.org/10.1016/j.ecns.2016.09.009

INACSL Standards Committee. (2016d, December). INACSL Standards of Best Practice: Simulation: Simulation design. *Clinical Simulation in Nursing, 12*, S5–S12. https://doi.org/10.1016/j.ecns.2016.09.005

INACSL Standards Committee. (2016e, December). INACSL Standards of Best Practice: Simulation: Simulation glossary. *Clinical Simulation in Nursing, 12*, S39–S47. https://doi.org/10.1016/j.ecns.2016.09.012

International Nursing Association for Clinical Simulation in Nursing (2011) Task Force. https://www.nursingsimulation.org/article/S1876-1399(13)00139-4/fulltext

Ironside, P. M., Jeffries, P. R., & Martin, A. (2009). Fostering patient safety competencies using multiple-patient simulation experiences. *Nursing Outlook, 57*(6), 332–337. doi:10.1016/j.outlook.2009.07.010

Issenberg, S. B., McGaghie, W. C., Petrusa, E. R., Gordon, D. L., & Scalese, R. J. (2005). Features and uses of high-fidelity medical simulations that lead to effective learning: A BEME systematic review. *Medical Teacher, 27*(1), 10–28. Retrieved from http://search.ebscohost.com/login.aspx?direct=true&db=rzh&AN=2005085405&site=ehost-live

Jeffries, P. R. (2005). A framework for designing, implementing and evaluating simulations used as teaching strategies in nursing. *Nursing Education Perspectives, 26*(2), 96–103. PMID: 15921126

Jeffries, P. R., & National League for Nursing, issuing body. (2016). *The NLN Jeffries simulation theory*. Philadelphia: Wolters Kluwer.

Jeffries, P. R., & Rizzolo, M. (2006). *Designing and implementing models for the innovative use of simulation to teach nursing care of ill adults and children: A national, multi-site, multi-method study*. National League for Nursing.

Jeffries, P. R., & Rogers, K. J. (2012). Theoretical framework for simulation design. In P. R. Jeffries (Ed.), *Simulation in nursing education: From conceptualization to evaluation* (2nd ed., pp. 25–42). National League for Nursing.

Johannesson, E., Olsson, M., Petersson, G., & Silén, C. (2010). Learning features in computer simulation skills training. *Nurse Education in Practice, 10*(5), 268–273. https://doi.org/10.1016/j.nepr.2009.11.018

Jones, A. L., Reese, C. E., & Shelton, D. P. (2014). NLN/Jeffries Simulation Framework state of the science project: The teacher construct. *Clinical Simulation in Nursing, 10*(7), 353–362. https://doi.org/10.1016/j.ecns.2013.10.008

Judd, B. K., Alison, J. A., Waters, D., & Gordon, C. J. (2016). Comparison of psychophysiological sress in physiotherapy students undertaking simulation and hospital-based clinical education. *Simulation in Healthcare: Journal of the Society for Medical Simulation, 11*(4), 271–277. doi: 10.1097/SIH.0000000000000155

Kaakinen, J., & Arwood, E. (2009). Systematic review of nursing simulation literature for use of learning theory. *International Journal of Nursing Education Scholarship, 6*(1), 1. https://doi.org/10.2202/1548-923X.1688

Kaplan, B. G., Abraham, C., & Gary, R. (2012). Effects of participation vs. observation of a simulation experience on testing outcomes: Implications for logistical planning for a school nursing. *International Journal of Nursing Education Scholarship, 9*(1), 1–15. Retrieved from http://search.ebscohost.com/login.aspx?direct=true&db=rzh&AN=2011630927&site=ehost-live

Kardong-Edgren, S., Starkweather, A. R., & Ward, L. D. (2008). The integration of simulation into a clinical foundations of nursing course: Student and faculty perspectives. *International Journal of Nursing Education Scholarship, 5*(1), 1–16. doi: 10.2202/1548-923X.1603

Karnath, B. M., Das Carlo, M., & Holden, M. D. (2004). A comparison of faculty-led small group learning in combination with computer-based instruction versus computer-based instruction alone on identifying simulated pulmonary sounds. *Teaching & Learning in Medicine, 16*(1), 23–27. Retrieved from http://search.ebscohost.com/login.aspx?direct=true&db=rzh&AN=2005028348&site=ehost-live

Kelly, M. A., Hager, P., & Gallagher, R. (2014). What matters most? Students' rankings of simulation components that contribute to clinical judgment. *Journal of Nursing Education, 53*(2), 97–101. https://doi.org/10.3928/01484834-20140122-08

Kennedy, C. C., Maldonado, F., & Cook, D. A. (2013). Simulation-based bronchoscopy training: Systematic review and meta-analysis. *Chest, 144*(1), 183–192. https://doi.org/10.1378/chest.12-1786

Kiat, T. K., Mei, T. Y., Nagammal, S., & Jonnie, A. (2007). A review of learners' experience with simulation based training in nursing. *Singapore Nursing Journal, 34*(4), 37–43. Retrieved from http://search.ebscohost.com/login.aspx?direct=true&db=rzh&AN=2009753282&site=ehost-live

Kirkpatrick, D. L. (1998). *Evaluating training programs: The four levels*. Bernett-Keehler.

Koskinen, L., Abdelhamid, P., & Likitalo, H. (2008). The simulation method for learning cultural awareness in nursing. *Diversity in Health & Social Care, 5*(1), 55–63. Retrieved from http://search.ebscohost.com/login.aspx?direct=true&db=rzh&AN=2009881225&site=ehost-live

LaFond, C. M., & Vincent, H. V. (2012). A critique of the National League for Nursing/Jeffries Simulation Framework. *Journal of Advanced Nursing, 69*(2), 465–480. https://doi.org/10.1111/j.1365-2648.2012.06048.x

Lane, C., & Rollnick, S. (2007). The use of simulated patients and role-play in communication skills training: A review of the literature to August 2005. *Patient Education & Counseling, 67*(1–2), 13–20. Retrieved from http://search.ebscohost.com/login.aspx?direct=true&db=rzh&AN=2009630289&site=ehost-live

Lapierre, A., Bouferguene, S., Gauvin-Lepage, J., Lavoie, P., & Arbour, C. (2020). Effectiveness of interprofessional manikin-based simulation training on teamwork among real teams during trauma resuscitation in adult emergency departments: A systematic review. *Simulation in Healthcare, 15*(6), 409–421. doi: 10.1097/SIH.0000000000000443

Lapkin, S., & Levett-Jones, T. (2011). A cost-utility analysis of medium vs. high-fidelity human patient simulation manikins in nursing education. *Journal of Clinical Nursing, 20*(23), 3543–3552. https://doi.org/10.1111/j.1365-2702.2011.03843.x

Leblanc, V. R., Regehr, C., Tavares, W., Scott, A. K., Macdonald, R., & King, K. (2012). The impact of stress on paramedic performance during simulated critical events. *Prehospital & Disaster Medicine, 27*(4), 369–374. Retrieved from http://search.ebscohost.com/login.aspx?direct=true&db=rzh&AN=20117 20637&site=ehost-live

Lee, Yu-Hsia, Lin, Shu-Chuan, Wang, Pao-Yu, & Mei-Hsiang, Lin. (2020). Objective structural clinical examination for evaluating learning efficacy of Cultural Competence Cultivation Programme for nurses. *BMC Nursing, 19*(1), 114. https://doi.org/10.1186/s12912-020-00500-3

LeFlore, J., & Anderson, M. (2009). Alternative educational models for interdisciplinary student teams. *Simulation in Healthcare, 4*, 135–142. https://doi.org/10.1097/SIH.0b013e318196f839

LeFlore, J., Anderson, M., Zielke, M., Nelson, K., Thomas, P., Hardee, G., & John, L. (2012). Can a virtual patient trainer teach student nurses how to save lives — Teaching nursing students about pediatric respiratory diseases. *Simulation in Healthcare, 7*, 10–17. https://doi.org/10.1097/SIH.0b013e31823652de

Leigh, G. T. (2008). High-fidelity patient simulation and nursing students' self-efficacy: A review of the literature. *International Journal of Nursing Education Scholarship, 5*(1), 17. Retrieved from http://search.ebscohost.com/login.aspx?direct=true&db=rzh&AN=2010044624&site=ehost-live

Leighton, K., & Scholl, K. (2009). Simulated codes: Understanding the response of undergraduate nursing students. *Clinical Simulation in Nursing, 5*(5), e187–e194. https://doi.org/10.1016/j.ecns.2009.05.058

Levett-Jones, T., & Lapkin, S. (2014). A systematic review of the effectiveness of simulation debriefing in health professional education. *Nurse Education Today, 34*(6), e58–e63. https://doi.org/10.1016/j.nedt.2013.09.020

Lineberry, M., Dev, P., Lane, H. C., & Talbot, T. B. (2018). Learner-adaptive educational technology for simulation in healthcare: Foundations and opportunities. *Simulation in Healthcare, 13*(3S Suppl 1), S21–S27 doi: 10.1097/SIH.0000000000000274

Lioce, L. (Ed.), Downing, D., Chang, T. P., Robertson, J. M., Anderson, M., Diaz, D. A., & Spain, A.E. (Assoc. Eds.) and the Terminology and Concepts Working Group. (2020, January). *Healthcare simulation dictionary – Second Edition*. Agency for Healthcare Research and Quality. AHRQ Publication No. 20-0019. https://doi.org/10.23970/simulationv2

Lucisano, K. E., & Talbot, L. A. (2012). Simulation training for advanced airway management for anesthesia and other healthcare providers: A systematic review. *AANA Journal, 80*(1), 25–31. Retrieved from http://search.ebscohost.com/login.aspx?direct=true&db=rzh&AN=2011485353&site=ehost-live

Maran, N. J., & Glavin, R. J. (2003). Low- to high-fidelity simulation — a continuum of medical education? *Medical Education, 37*, 22–28. https://doi.org/10.1046/j.1365-2923.37.s1.9.x

Marmol, M. T., Braga, F. T., Garbin, L. M., Moreli, L., dos Santos, C. B., & de Carvalho, E. C. (2012). Central catheter dressing in a simulator: The effects of tutor's assistance or self-learning tutorial. *Revista Latino-Americana De Enfermagem (RLAE), 20*(6), 1134–1141. doi: 10.1590/s0104-11692012000600016

Matos, F., & Raemer, D. (2013). Mixed-realism simulation of adverse event disclosure: An educational methodology and assessment instrument. *Simulation in Healthcare, 8*, 84–90. https://doi.org/10.1097/SIH.0b013e31827cbb27

McDermott, D. S. (2020, December). Prebriefing: A historical perspective and evolution of a model and strategy (know: do: teach). *Clinical Simulation in Nursing, 49*(C), 40–49. https://doi.org/10.1016/j.ecns.2020.05.005

McGaghie, W. C. (2008). Research opportunities in simulation-based medical education using deliberate practice. *Academic Emergency Medicine, 15*(11), 995–1001. Retrieved from http://search.ebscohost.com/login.aspx?direct=true&db=rzh&AN=2010386653&site=ehost-live

McGaghie, W. C., & Harris, I. B. (2018). Learning theory foundations of simulation-based mastery learning. *Simulation in Healthcare, 13*(3S Suppl 1), S15–S20. doi: 10.1097/SIH.0000000000000279

McGaghie, W. C., Issenberg, S. B., Barsuk, J. H., & Wayne, D. B. (2014). A critical review of simulation-based mastery learning with translational outcomes. *Medical Education, 48*(4), 375–385. https://doi.org/10.1111/medu.12391

McGaghie, W. C., Issenberg, S. B., Petrusa, E. R., & Scalese, R. J. (2006). Effect of practice on standardised learning outcomes in simulation-based medical education. *Medical Education, 40*(8), 792–797. Retrieved from http://search.ebscohost.com/login.aspx?direct=true&db=rzh&AN=2009257333&site=ehost-live

Meakim, C., Boese, T., Decker, S., Franklin, A. E., Gloe, D., Lioce, L., Sando, C. R., & Borum, J. C. (2013). Standards of Best Practice: Simulation standard I: Terminology. *Clinical Simulation in Nursing, 9*(6S), S3–S11. https://doi.org/10.1016/j.ecns.2013.04.001

Meyer, M., Connors, H., Hou, Q., & Gajewski, B. (2011). The effect of simulation on clinical performance: A junior nursing student clinical comparison study. *Simulation in Healthcare, 6*, 269–277. https://doi.org/10.1097/SIH.0b013e318223a048

Mills, B. W., Carter, O., Rudd, C., Claxton, L. A., Ross, N. P., & Strobel, N. A. (2016). Effects of low- versus high-fidelity simulations on the cognitive burden and performance of entry-level paramedicine students: A mixed-methods comparison trial using eye-tracking, continuous heart rate, difficulty rating scales, video observation and interviews. *Simulation in Healthcare, 11*(1), 10–18.

Montan, K. L., Hreckoviski, B., Dobson, B., Ortenwall, P., Montan, C., Khorram-Manesh, A., & Lennquist, L. (2014). Development and evaluation of a new simulation model for interactive training of the medical response to major incidents and disasters. *European Journal of Trauma and Emergency Surgery, 40*(4), 429–443. doi: 10.1007/s00068-013-0350-y

Mudumbai, S., Gaba, D., Boulet, J., Howard, S., & Davies, M. (2012). External validation of simulation-based assessments with other performance measures of third-year anesthesiology residents. *Simulation in Healthcare, 7*, 73–80. https://doi.org/10.1097/SIH.0b013e31823d018a

Nicholson, L. (2012). *The transformational learning process of nursing students during simulated clinical experiences*. D'Youville College. Doctoral dissertation. Retrieved from UMI number 3537521.

Norman, J. (2012). Systematic review of the literature on simulation in nursing education. *ABNF Journal, 23*(2), 24–28. Retrieved from http://search.ebscohost.com/login.aspx?direct=true&db=rzh&AN=2011552819&site=ehost-live

O'Donnell, J. M., Decker, S., Howard, V., Levett-Jones, T., & Miller, C. W. (2014). NLN/Jeffries Simulation Framework state of the science project: Simulation learning outcomes. *Clinical Simulation in Nursing, 10*(7), 373–382. https://doi.org/10.1016/j.ecns.2014.06.004

Onyura, B., Baker, L., Cameron, B., Friesen, F., & Leslie, K. (2016). Evidence for curricular and instructional design approaches in undergraduate medical education: An umbrella review. *Medical Teacher, 38*(2), 150–161. doi: 10.3109/0142159X.2015.1009019

Paige, J. B. (2014). *Simulation design characteristics: Perspectives held by nurse educators and nursing students*. University of Wisconsin–Milwaukee. Doctoral dissertation. Retrieved from UMI number 3614774.

Paige, J. B., & Morin, K. H. (2013). Simulation fidelity and cueing: A systematic review of the literature. *Clinical Simulation in Nursing, 9*(11), e481–e489. http://doi.org/10.1016/j.ecns.2013.01.001

Parker, B. C., & Myrick, F. (2012). The pedagogical ebb and flow of human patient simulation: Empowering through a process of fading support. *Journal of Nursing Education, 51*(7), 365–372. https://doi.org/10.3928/01484834-20120509-01

Parsh, B. (2010). Characteristics of effective simulated clinical experience instructors: Interviews with undergraduate nursing students. *Journal of Nursing Education, 49*(10), 569–572. https://doi.org/10.3928/01484834-20100730-04

Partin, J. L., Payne, T. A., & Slemmons, M. F. (2011). Students' perceptions of their learning experiences using high-fidelity simulation to teach concepts relative to obstetrics. *Nursing Education Perspectives, 32*(3), 186–188. https://doi.org/10.5480/1536-5026-32.3.186

Paskins, Z., & Peile, E. (2010). Final year medical students' views on simulation-based teaching: A comparison with the Best Evidence Medical Education systematic review. *Medical Teacher, 32*(7), 569–577. https://doi.org/10.3109/01421590903544710

Perretta, J. S., Duval-Arnould, J., Poling, S., Sullivan, N., Jeffers, J., Farrow, L., Shilkofski, N. A., Brown, K. M., & Hunt, E. A. (2020). Best practices and theoretical foundations for simulation instruction using rapid-cycle deliberate practice. *Simulation in Healthcare, 15*(5), 356–362. doi: 10.1097/SIH.0000000000000433

Prion, S., & Haerling, K. A. (2017). Making sense of methods and measurements: Linking simulation to patient outcomes. *Clinical Simulation in Nursing, 13*(6), 291–292. https://doi.org/10.1016/j.ecns.2017.01.007

Pusic, M., Boutis, K., & McGaghie, W. C. (2018). Role of scientific theory in simulation education research. *Simulation in Healthcare, 13*(3S Suppl 1), S7–S14. doi: 10.1097/SIH.0000000000000282

Ravert, P. (2002). An integrative review of computer-based simulation in the education process. *CIN: Computers, Informatics, Nursing, 20*(5), 203–208. doi: 10.1097/00024665-200209000-00013

Rezmer, J., Begaz, T., Treat, R., & Tews, M. (2011). Impact of group size on the effectiveness of a resuscitation simulation curriculum for medical students. *Teaching & Learning in Medicine, 23*(3), 251–255. https://doi.org/10.1080/10401334.2011.586920

Rogers, B., Baker, K. A., & Franklin, A. E. (2020, December). Learning outcomes of the observer role in nursing simulation: A scoping review. *Clinical Simulation in Nursing, 49*(C), 81–89. https://doi.org/10.1016/j.ecns.2020.06.003

Roh, Y. S., & Lim, E. J. (2014). Pre-course simulation as a predictor of satisfaction with an emergency nursing clinical course. *International Journal of Nursing Education Scholarship, 11*(1), 1–8. https://doi.org/10.1515/ijnes-2013-0083

Rosen, M. A., Hunt, E. A., Pronovost, P. J., Federowicz, M. A., & Weaver, S. J. (2012). In situ simulation in continuing education for the health care professions: A systematic review. *Journal of Continuing Education in the Health Professions, 32*(4), 243–254. https://doi.org/10.1002/chp.21152

Rossler, K. L., Hardin, K., & Taylor, J. (2020, December). Teaching interprofessional socialization and collaboration to nurses transitioning into critical care. *Clinical Simulation in Nursing, 49*(C), 9–15. https://doi.org/10.1016/j.ecns.2020.03.012

Rourke, L., Schmidt, M., & Garga, N. (2010). Theory-based research of high fidelity simulation use in nursing education: A review of the literature. *International Journal of Nursing Education Scholarship, 7*(1), 14. https://doi.org/10.2202/1548-923X.1965

Salas, E. (2016). Reporting guidelines for health care simulation research: Where is the learning? *Simulation in Healthcare, 11*(4), 249.

Santomauro, C. M., Hill, A., McCurdie, T., & McGlashan, H. L. (2020). Improving the quality of evaluation data in simulation-based healthcare improvement projects: A practitioner's guide to choosing and using published measurement tools. *Simulation in Healthcare, 15*(5), 341–355. doi: 10.1097/SIH.0000000000000442

Scaringe, J. G., Chen, D., & Ross, D. (2002). The effects of augmented sensory feedback precision on the acquisition and retention of a simulated chiropractic task. *Journal of Manipulative & Physiological Therapeutics, 25*(1), 34–41. Retrieved from http://search.ebscohost.com/login.aspx?direct=true&db=rzh&AN=2002057675&site=ehost-live

Schlairet, M. C., & Fenster, M. J. (2012). Dose and sequence of simulation and direct care experiences among beginning nursing students: A pilot study. *Journal of Nursing Education, 51*(12), 668–675. https://doi.org/10.3928/01484834-20121005-03

Schwartz, L. R., Fernandez, R., Kouyoumjian, S. R., Jones, K. A., & Compton, S. (2007). A randomized comparison trial of case-based learning versus human patient simulation in medical student education. *Academic Emergency Medicine, 14*(2), 130–137. Retrieved from http://search.ebscohost.com/login.aspx?direct=true&db=rzh&AN=2009507277&site=ehost-live

Seaton, P., Levett-Jones, T., Cant, R., Cooper, S., Kelly, M. A., McKenna, L., Ng, L., & Bogossian, F. (2019). Exploring the extent to which simulation-based education addresses contemporary patient safety priorities: A scoping review. *Collegian (Royal College of Nursing, Australia), 26*(1), 194–203. https://doi.org/10.1016/j.colegn.2018.04.006

Shanks, D., Brydges, R., den Brok, W., Nair, P., & Hatala, R. (2013). Are two heads better than one? Comparing dyad and self-regulated learning in simulation training. *Medical Education, 47*(12), 1215–1222. https://doi.org/10.1111/medu.12284

Shinnick, M. A., Woo, M., & Evangelista, L. S. (2012). Predictors of knowledge gains using simulation in the education of prelicensure nursing students. *Journal of Professional Nursing, 28*(1), 41–47. https://doi.org/10.1016/j.profnurs.2011.06.006

Smith, S. J., & Roehrs, C. J. (2009). High-fidelity simulation: Factors correlated with nursing student satisfaction and self-confidence. *Nursing Education Perspectives, 30*(2), 74–78. PMID: 19476068

Smithburger, P., Kane-Gill, S., Ruby, C., & Seybert, M. (2012). Comparing effectiveness of 3 learning strategies: Simulation-based learning, problem-based learning, and standardized patients. *Simulation in Healthcare, 7*, 141–146. https://doi.org/10.1097/SIH.0b013e31823ee24d

Solli, H., Haukedal, T. A., Husebo, S. E., & Reierson, I. Å. (2020). The art of balancing: The facilitator's role in briefing in simulation-based learning from the perspective of nursing students — a qualitative study. *BMC Nursing, 19*(1), 99. https://doi.org/10.1016/j.ecns.2009.10.003

Stegmann, K., Pilz, F., Siebeck, M., & Fischer, F. (2012). Vicarious learning during simulations: Is it more effective than hands-on training? *Medical Education, 46*(10), 1001–1008. https://doi.org/10.1111/j.1365-2923.2012.04344.x

Tiffen, J., Corbridge, S., Shen, B. C., & Robinson, P. (2011). Patient simulator for teaching heart and lung assessment skills to advanced practice nursing students. *Clinical Simulation in Nursing, 7*(3), e91–e97. https://doi.org/10.1016/j.ecns.2009.10.003

Tosterud, R., Hedelin, B., & Hall-Lord, M. L. (2013). Nursing students' perceptions of high and low-fidelity simulation used as learning methods. *Nursing Education in Practice, 13*, 262–270. doi: 10.1016/j.nepr.2013.02.002

Trokan-Mathison, N. (2013). *Using simulation to foster the quality and safety education for nurses competencies in associate degree nursing students*. Capella University. Doctoral dissertation. Retrieved from UMI number 3597401.

Tyerman, J., Luctkar-Flude, M., Graham, L., Coffey, S., & Olsen-Lynch, E. (2019, February). A systematic review of health care presimulation preparation and briefing effectiveness. *Clinical Simulation in Nursing,*

27(C), 12–25. https://doi.org/10.1016/j.ecns.2018.11.002

van Soeren, M., Devlin-Cop, S., MacMillan, K., Baker, L., Egan-Lee, E., & Reeves, S. (2011). Simulated interprofessional education: An analysis of teaching and learning processes. *Journal of Interprofessional Care, 25*(6), 434–440. https://doi.org/10.3109/13561820.2011.592229

Verkuyl, M., Lapum, J. L., St-Amant, O., Hughes, M., Romaniuk, D., & McCulloch, T. (2020). Exploring debriefing combinations after a virtual simulation. *Clinical Simulation in Nursing, 40*(C), 36–42. https://doi.org/10.1016/j.ecns.2019.12.002

Verkuyl, M., Richie, S., Cahuas, D., Rowland, C., Ndondo, M., Larcina, T., & Mack, K. (2020). Exploring self-debriefing plus group-debriefing: A focus group study. *Clinical Simulation in Nursing, 43*(C), 3–9. https://doi.org/10.1016/j.ecns.2020.03.007

Walsh, C. M., Sherlock, M. E., Ling, S. C., & Carnahan, H. (2012). Virtual reality simulation training for health professions trainees in gastrointestinal endoscopy. *Cochrane Database of Systematic Reviews*, (6). Retrieved from http://search.ebscohost.com/login.aspx?direct=true&db=rzh&AN=2011632632&site=ehost-live

Waxman, K. T. (2010). The development of evidence-based clinical simulation scenarios: Guidelines for nurse educators. *Journal of Nursing Education, 49*(1), 29–35. https://doi.org/10.3928/01484834-20090916-07

Wilbanks, B. A., McMullan, S., Watts, P. I., White, T., & Moss, J. (2020, May). Comparison of videofacilitated reflective practice and faculty-led debriefings. *Clinical Simulation in Nursing, 42*(C), 1–7. https://doi.org/10.1016/j.ecns.2019.12.007

Wong, F., Cheung, S., Chung, L., Chan, K., Chan, A., To, T., & Wong, M. (2008). Framework for adopting a problem-based learning approach in a simulated clinical setting. *Journal of Nursing Education, 47*(11), 508–514. https://doi.org/10.3928/01484834-20081101-11

Wright, M., Segall, N., Hobbs, G., Phillips-Bute, B., Maynard, L., & Taekman, J. (2013). Standardized assessment for evaluation of team skills: Validity and feasibility. *Simulation in Healthcare, 8*, 292–303. https://doi.org/10.1097/SIH.0b013e318290a022

Yang, H., Thompson, C., & Bland, M. (2012). Effect of improving the realism of simulated clinical judgment tasks on nurses' overconfidence and under confidence: Evidence from a comparative confidence calibration analysis. *International Journal of Nursing Studies, 49*(12), 1505–1511. https://doi.org/10.1016/j.ijnurstu.2012.08.005

Yuan, H. B., Williams, B. A., & Fang, J. B. (2012). The contribution of high-fidelity simulation to nursing students' confidence and competence: A systematic review. *International Nursing Review, 59*(1), 26–33. https://doi.org/10.1111/j.1466-7657.2011.00964.x

Yuan, H. B., Williams, B. A., Fang, J. B., & Ye, Q. H. (2012). A systematic review of selected evidence on improving knowledge and skills through high-fidelity simulation. *Nurse Education Today, 32*(3), 294–298. https://doi.org/10.1016/j.nedt.2011.07.010

Zulkosky, K. D. (2012). Simulation use in the classroom: Impact on knowledge acquisition, satisfaction and self-confidence. *Clinical Simulation in Nursing, 8*(1), e25–e33. https://doi.org/10.1016/j.ecns.2010.06.003

3

NLN Jeffries Simulation Theory: Brief Narrative Description

Pamela R. Jeffries, PhD, RN, FAAN, ANEF
Beth Rodgers, PhD, RN, FAAN
Katie Anne Haerling (Adamson), PhD, RN, CHSE

INTRODUCTION

Based on the thorough synthesis of the literature and discussion among simulation researchers and leaders, the NLN Jeffries Simulation Framework (2005, 2007, 2012) is now referred to as the NLN Jeffries Simulation theory with a few minor changes within the conceptual illustration. In this chapter, the concepts of this theory are briefly described to provide more clarity and to explain Figure 3.1, as well as the new NLN Jeffries Simulation theory.

CONTEXT

Contextual factors such as *circumstances* and *setting* impact every aspect of the simulation and are an important starting point in designing or evaluating simulation. The **context** may include the place (academic vs. practice; *in situ* vs. lab) and the overarching purpose of the simulation; for example, whether the simulation is for evaluation or instructional purposes.

BACKGROUND

Within this context, the **background** includes the goal(s) of the simulation and specific expectations or benchmarks that influence the **design** of the simulation. The theoretical perspective for the specific **simulation experience** and how the simulation fits within the larger curriculum are all important elements of the background and inform the simulation design and implementation. Finally, the background of a simulation includes resources such as time and equipment, as well as how these resources will be allocated.

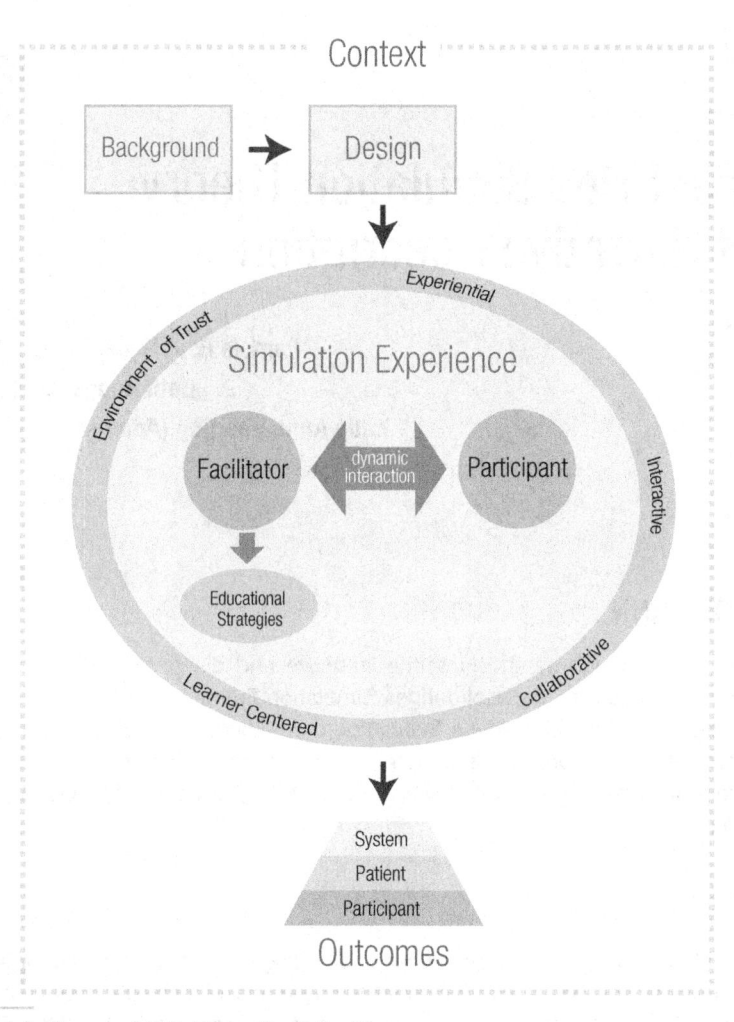

FIGURE 3.1 Diagram of NLN Jeffries Simulation Theory.

DESIGN

Outside of and preceding the actual simulation experience are specific elements that make up the simulation design. Although some elements of the simulation design may be changed during implementation of the simulation experience, there are aspects of the design that need to be considered in preparation for the simulation experience. The design includes the specific learning objectives that guide the development or selection of activities and scenario(s) with appropriate content and problem-solving complexity. Elements of physical and conceptual fidelity — including decisions about equipment, moulage (physical), and appropriate, predetermined **facilitator** responses to **participants**' interventions (conceptual) — are established as part of the simulation design. Participant and observer roles (including whether or not videography will be used), progression of activities, and briefing/debriefing strategies are all established as part of the simulation design.

SIMULATION EXPERIENCE

The simulation experience is characterized by an environment that is experiential, interactive, collaborative, and learner centered. This environment requires the establishment of trust; both the facilitator and participant share responsibility for maintaining this environment. They enhance the quality of the simulation experience through "buying-in" to the authenticity of the experience and suspending disbelief. This helps promote engagement and psychological fidelity within the simulation experience (Harder, 2018; Leighton & Scholl, 2009; van Soeren et al., 2011).

FACILITATOR AND EDUCATIONAL STRATEGIES

Within this simulation experience is a dynamic interaction between the facilitator and the participant. The literature about the characteristics these individuals bring to the simulation experience and how they affect the simulation experience is extensive. Facilitator attributes include (but are not limited to) skill, educational techniques, and preparation (Parker & Myrick, 2012; Parsh, 2010; Solli et al., 2020). The facilitator responds to emerging participant needs during the simulation experience by adjusting educational strategies such as altering the planned progression and timing of activities and providing appropriate feedback in the form of cues (during) and debriefing (toward the end) of the simulation experience (Ali & Musallam, 2018; Gantt et al., 2018; Wilbanks et al., 2020).

PARTICIPANT

Participant attributes also affect the simulation learning experience. The literature describes attributes that are innate to the participant such as age (Fenske et al., 2013), gender (Diez et al., 2013), level of anxiety (Beischel, 2011; Leblanc et al., 2012), and self-confidence (Jeffries & Rogers, 2012) as well as modifiable attributes such as preparedness for the simulation (Beischel, 2011). Many elements of the simulation design such as role assignment affect individual participants and may impact their learning experience (Kaplan et al., 2012).

OUTCOMES

Finally, outcomes of the simulation may be separated into three areas: participant, patient (or care recipient), and system outcomes. The literature largely focuses on participant outcomes including reaction (satisfaction, self-confidence), learning (changes in knowledge, skills, attitudes), and behavior (how learning transfers to the clinical environment) (McGaghie & Harris, 2018). However, there is emerging literature about outcomes of simulation covering health outcomes of patients or care recipients whose caregivers were trained using simulation and organizational/system outcomes of simulation, including studies about cost-effectiveness and changes of practice (Prion & Haerling, 2014; Seaton et al., 2019).

Figure 3.1 depicts outcomes in a triangular format based on the hierarchy of participant, patient, and system outcomes as defined and extracted from the body of literature found on simulation outcomes.

References

Alhaj Ali, A., & Musallam, E. (2018, March). Debriefing quality evaluation in nursing simulation-based education: An integrative review. *Clinical Simulation in Nursing, 16*, 15–24. https://doi.org/10.1016/j.ecns.2017.09.009

Beischel, K. P. (2011). Variables affecting learning in a simulation experience: A mixed methods study. *Western Journal of Nursing Research, 35*(2), 226–247. doi: 10.1177/0193945911408444

Diez, N., Rodriguez-Diez, M., Nagore, D., Fernandez, S., Ferrer, M., & Beunza, J. (2013). A randomized trial of cardiopulmonary resuscitation training for medical students: Voice advisory mannequin compared to guidance provided by an instructor. *Simulation in Healthcare: The Journal of the Society for Simulation in Healthcare, 8*, 234–241. https://doi.org/10.1097/SIH.0b013e31828e7196

Fenske, C. L., Harris, M. A., Aebersold, M. L., & Hartman, L. S. (2013). Perception versus reality: A comparative study of the clinical judgment skills of nurses during a simulated activity. *Journal of Continuing Education in Nursing, 44*(9), 399–405. https://doi.org/10.3928/00220124-20130701-67

Gantt, L. T., Overton, S. H., Avery, J., Swanson, M., & Elhammoumi, C. V. (2018, April). Comparison of debriefing methods and learning outcomes in human patient simulation. *Clinical Simulation in Nursing, 17*, 7–13. https://doi.org/10.1016/j.ecns.2017.11.012

Harder, N. (2018). Dealing with the fidelity of simulation-based learning. *Clinical Simulation in Nursing, 25*, 20–21. https://doi.org/10.1016/j.ecns.2018.10.004

Jeffries, P. R. (2005). A framework for designing, implementing, and evaluating simulations used as teaching strategies in nursing. *Nursing Education Perspectives, 26*(2), 96–103. doi: 10.1043/1536-5026(2005)026<0096:AFWFDI>2.0.CO;2

Jeffries, P. R. (Ed.). (2007). *Simulation in nursing education: From conceptualization to evaluation*. National League for Nursing.

Jeffries, P. R. (Ed.). (2012). *Simulation in nursing education: From conceptualization to evaluation* (2nd ed.). National League for Nursing.

Jeffries, P. R., & Rogers, K. J. (2012). Theoretical framework for simulation design. In P. R. Jeffries (Ed.), *Simulation in nursing education: From conceptualization to evaluation* (2nd ed., pp. 25–42). National League for Nursing.

Kaplan, B. G., Abraham, C., & Gary, R. (2012). Effects of participation vs. observation of a simulation experience on testing outcomes: Implications for logistical planning for a school of nursing. *International Journal of Nursing Education Scholarship, 9*(1), 1–15. Retrieved from http://search.ebscohost.com/login.aspx?direct=true&db=rzh&AN=2011630927&site=ehost-live

Leblanc, V. R., Regehr, C., Tavares, W., Scott, A. K., Macdonald, R., & King, K. (2012). The impact of stress on paramedic performance during simulated critical events. *Prehospital & Disaster Medicine, 27*(4), 369–374. Retrieved from http://search.ebscohost.com/login.aspx?direct=true&db=rzh&AN=2011720637&site=ehost-live

Leighton, K., & Scholl, K. (2009). Simulated codes: Understanding the response of undergraduate nursing students. *Clinical Simulation in Nursing, 5*(5), e187–e194. https://doi.org/10.1016/j.ecns.2009.05.058

McGaghie, W. C., & Harris, I. B. (2018). Learning theory foundations of simulation-based mastery learning. *Simulation in Healthcare*, *13*(3S Suppl 1), S15–S20. doi: 10.1097/SIH.0000000000000279

Parker, B. C., & Myrick, F. (2012). The pedagogical ebb and flow of human patient simulation: Empowering through a process of fading support. *Journal of Nursing Education*, *51*(7), 365–372. https://doi.org/10.3928/01484834-20120509-01

Parsh, B. (2010). Characteristics of effective simulated clinical experience instructors: Interviews with undergraduate nursing students. *Journal of Nursing Education*, *49*(10), 569–572. https://doi.org/10.3928/01484834-20100730-04

Prion, S., & Haerling, K. A. (2014). Making sense of methods and measurements: Linking simulation to patient outcomes. *Clinical Simulation in Nursing*, *13*(6), 291–292. doi:10.1016/j.ecns.2014.07.010

Seaton, P., Levett-Jones, T., Cant, R., Cooper, S., Kelly, M. A., McKenna, L., Ng, L., & Bogossian, F. (2019). Exploring the extent to which simulation-based education addresses contemporary patient safety priorities: A scoping review. *Collegian (Royal College of Nursing, Australia)*, *26*(1), 194–203. https://doi.org/10.1016/j.colegn.2018.04.006

Solli, H., Haukedal, T. A., Husebo, S. E., & Reierson, I. Å. (2020). The art of balancing: The facilitator's role in briefing in simulation-based learning from the perspective of nursing students — a qualitative study. *BMC Nursing*, *19*(1), 99. doi: 10.1186/s12912-020-00493-z

Wilbanks, B. A., McMullan, S., Watts, P. I., White, T., & Moss, J. (2020, May). Comparison of video-facilitated reflective practice and faculty-led debriefings. *Clinical Simulation in Nursing*, *42*(C), 1–7. https://doi.org/10.1016/j.ecns.2019.12.007

van Soeren, M., Devlin-Cop, S., MacMillan, K., Baker, L., Egan-Lee, E., & Reeves, S. (2011). Simulated interprofessional education: An analysis of teaching and learning processes. *Journal of Interprofessional Care*, *25*(6), 434–440. https://doi.org/10.3109/13561820.2011.592229

4

Guidelines in Using the Theory in Nursing Education, Practice, and Research

Beth Rodgers, PhD, RN, FAAN

INTRODUCTION

Theory is a vital aspect of nursing and, in general, a vital aspect of any activity. Most nurses, however, receive only a rudimentary exposure to theory, if any exposure at all. Around the mid-20th century, nursing students received considerable exposure to an array of "nursing theories" in ways that may or may not have prompted appreciation for or interest in theoretical thinking. Over time, the amount of attention given to theory has decreased, partly due to the need to devote precious time in curricula to learning the increasingly complex work of nursing. The decrease in attention may also have been driven by those earlier introductions to theory which did not always develop interest or appreciation for the importance of theory in the science and work of nurses. As a result of limited, and later diminished, attention to theory, a large number of nurses do not have the understanding or skills needed to use and evaluate theory effectively in their own work (Rodgers, 2005).

The work of nurses is strengthened considerably when there is a solid understanding of theory and knowledge of how theory contributes to that work. Another important outcome of the understanding and, especially, use of theory in doing work in an area is that it can facilitate progress in growing knowledge in an area of interest. The National League for Nursing (NLN) Jeffries Simulation theory provides a solid, research-based foundation to guide simulation experiences, and nurses need to understand how to make effective use of this important work. Such understanding can provide nurse educators with assistance in creating and evaluating constructive simulation experiences but also in contributing to an expanded body of simulation science.

Theory is not just an elusive, abstract description of a state of something; it can also be a very practical and useful aid. In very simple terms, theory can be thought of as a guide. Theory tells the person working with the theory how to get to a particular place, what to expect on arrival, what it would be wise to do while there, and what are the best ways to get around. The concepts presented in a theory point out important considerations, and stated relationships are like the roads between those points of interest.

Theory also points out things to watch for as well as provides some ideas of what will happen if a particular path is followed. A good guide also can steer the user away from pitfalls by making clear the limitations of a particular path or areas in which not enough is known. In the case of theory, there also usually are good clues for what needs to be developed further or what has not yet been fully explored.

THEORY IN ACTION: SIMULATION EDUCATION

In regard to knowledge — in this case, knowledge of simulation — theory serves to organize what is known and group information into key concepts. Theory shows how the concepts of the theory are connected and provides insight into how a change in one area may lead to another change in some other component. Theory offers a convenient package of knowledge that enables knowledge to be applied and transferred across a variety of different situations. Theory of simulation offers a foundation of knowledge that can be used in confronting or planning any simulation experience (Jeffries & Rodgers, 2020).

Without theory, each experience might be seen as an isolated case. If the idea of working from a theoretical foundation seems unfamiliar, it may be helpful to recognize that theoretical thinking exists whenever knowledge is transferred from one situation to another. Such theory is not always stated or acknowledged directly, however, but can remain implicit. This aspect of theory often goes unrecognized. When there is thinking along the lines of "I want students to learn a particular thing, so I'm going to try this approach," there is theoretical thinking behind that decision. Such statements are based on ideas about the nature of learning and the relationships among certain actions and the outcomes they are expected to produce. Theoretical thinking always is present in some form, even when those relationships are very general or limited in scope. Using a specific, delineated, and well-supported theory can help to make such thinking explicit, provide explanations of how and why decisions were made, and provide even greater support for the delivery of quality simulations.

Making the theoretical basis for simulation work clear benefits the work of nurses and the development of the theory in other ways. A theoretical foundation provides a shared point of reference across settings and across disciplines. It provides a common point of view and language to enable collaboration and also to create a robust network for continuing development of that theory. When a theory is applied and evaluated across multiple contexts and varied applications, there is greatly increased potential for continuing development of the theory.

The NLN Jeffries Simulation theory works as previously described in the same way as other theories. It provides information about what needs to be considered in preparing and delivering simulation, how to develop and deliver the simulation, and what to consider for outcomes. It elucidates the roles of the people involved in any simulation experience and points to areas in which outcomes can be measured. Without a theoretical foundation, nurses working in the area of simulation may easily overlook critical components of the simulation process. Major pitfalls can be avoided by using the theory for guidance in creating simulations, taking advantage of its strong conceptual foundation and extensive research support.

As an example, a common trend in simulation is to focus on the simulation case or experience itself, the facilitator and participant, and the specific situation being addressed. The theory, however, draws attention to background and contextual information that also are critical in any simulation and which may be overlooked by a focus on the more immediate concerns associated with immersion in an actual simulation experience. The theory also points out that outcomes can be observed on multiple levels, rather than on the mere tendency to look at an individual participant's or learner's objectives.

USING THEORY TO DEVELOP THEORY

Not only is it important to use theory to guide the development and delivery of simulation for learning, but it is important to evaluate that use and contribute to further development of the theory. The state of development of a theory will affect just how much information is provided and the quality of that information. Theory is never complete or perfect, and the situations to which they apply can be expanded. Although theory provides an important guide, it also can limit what is explored. Theory should be applied in a way that maximizes the benefit of using the theory to the benefit of simulation experiences, but not in a way that restricts noticing other conditions or questions that arise. The theory provides a solid focal point and foundation for simulation, but also can be expanded and strengthened through consideration of other aspects that are identified in the process of developing and delivering simulations. Theory needs to be continually applied and tested, and results used to further validate and refine the theory. With repeated use and testing, the theory will yield an increasingly more robust and detailed guide for future use. Those using theory can benefit not only from the guidance the theory offers for their own work, but they can contribute to continuing development of the theory.

An example of how theory can guide development and delivery of simulation is evident in looking at a common situation in educational settings. The focus of simulation often is on what actually happens during the simulated experience. Educators will spend a lot of time selecting a case to use for the simulation, deciding what should happen during the simulation or what are the key learning indicators, adapting the simulation to the program and curricular needs and resources, and developing a script for preparing the participant/learner prior to starting the simulation. A large portion of simulation time commonly is devoted to debriefing. This approach has yielded many positive results and has shown good learning outcomes for simulation in a variety of situations.

The theory shows that there are many elements that may be overlooked by a focus specifically on the simulation experience. Following the NLN Jeffries Simulation theory, the nurse can see that a quality simulation actually begins with consideration of context, including issues related to background and design. The simulation experience involves numerous aspects related to the participant and the facilitator, including the active employment of educational strategies by the facilitator. Without a theoretical perspective that calls attention to these important aspects, delineated in the later description of the theory, a less comprehensive approach to the situation results. It is comparable to preparing a course on a topic and thinking in terms of "this is what I want to tell the students," an approach that delivers content, but fails to consider the many aspects of learning beyond content delivery. Presenting a variety of content to students probably will lead to some learning, but it is clear from learning theories that a thoughtful approach that starts with clear learning objectives provides a far better learning experience.

THEORETICAL PERSPECTIVES IN RESEARCH

Simulation theory works in the same way as it directs the educator to consider a variety of elements that might otherwise be overlooked. Questions such as the following should be considered: What setting is this in? What is the purpose of the simulation? What are the goals to be accomplished and why simulation rather than some other approach? In terms of the design, what type of simulation should be provided? How do I ensure fidelity? What prior experiences have students encountered that are relevant to the experience? What preparation should be provided – how much detail? Should they have readings in advance or should they encounter the simulated experience in a manner more comparable to a real life scenario where there may be little or no information available? The specific elements of the simulation are highlighted as well, along with consideration for the participants as individuals or as a group. How does the educator direct the simulation? What facilitation strategies and feedback strategies should be used? What can the educator expect as a result of these decisions, based on what is already known through research using this theory? How is learning evaluated? What other outcomes might be expected? How should the simulation be managed overall to ensure an effective learning experience including elements of fidelity, time on task, and resources?

These are just a few of the questions that the educator is prompted to consider when using the theory to develop and implement simulation activities. In addition to the benefits of this guidance from the theory, the nurse educator also gains insight into how simulation activities might be studied and can share these results with others. A decision made regarding an aspect of the design, for example, as prompted by the theory, creates a situation for applying and expanding an aspect of the theory. That information can be shared with others, whether evaluated through formal research or by way of experiential reports of successes and insights gained. The end of this monograph provides additional information about research areas and emerging trends, as well as ideas for future research to continue development and strengthening of the theory.

The NLN Jeffries Simulation theory has a broad range of use across multiple levels of learners and varied disciplines. It can be used with entry level learners and with those preparing for advanced levels of practice and certification. Simulation can be oriented primarily toward learning or for evaluation purposes. The NLN Jeffries Simulation theory has been used in a variety of settings and disciplines including with international contexts and student groups.

Working from the foundation of a well-established, shared theoretical perspective with substantial research support offers tremendous advantage to the nurse educator and colleagues. It provides a valuable guide for development of quality simulation learning environments and experiences, promotes a comprehensive view of the how and why of simulation, and facilitates effective evaluation of outcomes. It offers a shared point of reference for interdisciplinary and interprofessional collaboration and common ways of conceptualizing aspects of simulation work. It also offers an important opportunity for a feedback loop for promoting continuing refinement and expansion of this important aspect of simulation knowledge and the use of simulation to improve education and practice.

References

Jeffries, P., & Rodgers, B. (2020). The NLN Jeffries Simulation theory. In P. R. Jeffries (Ed.), *Simulation in nursing education: From conceptualization to evaluation* (3rd ed., n.p.). Wolters Kluwer.

Rodgers, B. L. (2005). *Development of nursing knowledge*. Lippincott, Williams, and Wilkins.

5

From Vision Statement to Reality: Educational Best Practices Across the Curriculum: EPQ-C

Susan Gross Forneris, PhD, RN, CNE, CHSE-A, FAAN
Bette Mariani, PhD, RN, FAAN, ANEF
Amy Daniels, PhD, RN, CHSE
Cynthia Sherraden Bradley, PhD, RN, CNE, CHSE
Mary K. Fey, PhD, RN, CHSE-A, FAAN, ANEF

INTRODUCTION

The National Academy of Medicine (2020) *Future of Nursing 2020–2030* highlights the current and future challenges for health care. The report also addresses the current state of the science and technology informs how we assess the nursing profession's ability to meet the demands of the health care system in 2020 and beyond. The nature of education required to prepare professional nurses continues to challenge nursing education with emphasis on meeting the needs of diverse learners as we refocus nursing curricula to prepare our next generation of learners.

HISTORICAL PERSPECTIVE ON BEST PRACTICES IN TEACHING AND LEARNING

With the widespread adoption of simulation as a teaching-learning methodology following the 2003 to 2006 National League for Nursing (NLN)/Laerdal simulation study in nursing education, the need to set standards for the practice was recognized. The board of directors (BOD) of the International Nursing Association for Clinical Simulation and Learning (INACSL) published the first Standards of Best Practice: Simulation[SM] (SOBP) in 2011 (INACSL BOD, 2011). Updates continue to be made to the standards with the latest evidence. The SOBP provide a sound evidence base for educators using simulation, and offer guidance on terminology, simulation design, professional integrity of participants, participant objectives and outcomes, facilitation, debriefing, participant evaluation, Simulation-Enhanced Interprofessional Education (Sim-IPE), and operations (INACSL Standards Committee, 2016). Created by an interprofessional, international group of simulation educators, the SOBP set the bar for high-quality simulation-based education. Embedded throughout the Standards is the call for theoretically based practices in the design and delivery of simulation-based educational experiences.

In 2015, the NLN published the Vision Statement: A Vision for Teaching with Simulation (NLN, 2015a) that advocated for the use of simulation as a way to foster clinical reasoning skills as students learn in a realistic clinical context. The Vision Statement advocated the increased use of simulation to prepare students for practice. It recognized the transformational nature of learning in simulation because of the unique opportunity it presented for situated cognition. The Vision Statement also encouraged the use of the NLN Jeffries Simulation Framework (Jeffries, 2005), later known as the NLN Jeffries Simulation theory (Jeffries et al., 2015), as the theoretical foundation for research in simulation use and efficacy.

Since that work, simulation has been education's *disruptor* or "Trojan Horse" (Waxman et al., 2019). Simulation frameworks and theories have emerged and accompanied the SOBP (2016) to outline what it means to deliver best practice in teaching and learning (Cowperthwait, 2020; Jones & Alinier, 2015; Nestel & Bearman, 2015). These emerging theories are grounded in evidence, supporting simulation as an effective evidence-based strategy for teaching-learning. Nursing education leaders are now asking important questions about clinical learning and examining previously unchallenged assumptions about best practices, such as the primacy of clinical experiences as a pathway to developing reflective clinical practitioners.

Simulation as an active teaching-learning strategy has pushed the boundaries of experiential learning and classroom learning in higher education. Educators are now involved in thoughtful planning in the design of learning spaces and how the learning space engages learners individually and collaboratively. Nurse educators are now recognizing the importance of creating and implementing teaching methodologies that replace inactive, traditional lecture-based classroom learning environments.

Neuroscience research informs these new teaching methodologies, providing insight on how the brain works. The evidence suggests that once-tested and proven strategies are not working with today's learners (Alexander et al., 2019; Argawal, 2019). Simulation started us on that trajectory with less emphasis on providing the learner with the *content* and more emphasis and opportunities to *use the content* (Forneris & Fey, 2020); hence, brain-based learning is changing the face of education today (Cardoza, 2011; Doyle & Zakrajsek, 2019; Pan & Rickard, 2018; Weidman & Baker, 2015).

While some of these teaching strategies may be unlike our traditional experiences of classroom lecture, the common thread is the educator's assessment of *how the content is being processed in the learner's brain*. Earlier work in educational best practices in teaching and learning continue to inform neuroscience and have been foundational to active learning strategies, like simulation and debriefing, that are used today (Chickering & Gamson, 1987).

TOWARD A CONTEMPORARY APPROACH TO TEACHING AND LEARNING ACROSS THE CURRICULUM

Chickering and Gamson (1987) identified seven guiding principles for educators and learners to improve teaching and learning in higher education. These principles were guided by 50 years of research that examined how educators teach, how learners best learn, and how learners and educators interact and communicate. Each individual guideline can be implemented with positive improvements; when implemented collectively, the guidelines support the constructs of activity, cooperation, diversity, expectations, interaction, and responsibility (Chickering & Gamson, 1987). These constructs are integral to engaged teaching and learning and can be applied to all content across undergraduate education. A key driver for developing these guiding principles (Chickering & Gamson, 1987) was to prepare learners to understand and interact with "real life" by learning how to process and apply the knowledge, attitudes, and skills learned in higher education.

Intentionally aligning teaching practice with the seven principles of good educational practices (Chickering & Gamson, 1987) supports a collaborative learning environment that facilitates engaged learning. Specifically, these principles are to encourage contact between learners and educators, develop reciprocity and cooperation among learners, give prompt feedback, use active learning techniques, and respect diverse talents and ways of learning (Chickering & Gamson, 1987). As higher education curricular trends have adopted more active learning strategies, these principles have become not only a guide for educators in developing learning experiences, but also an expectation of learners as they prepare for more meaningful activities. In nursing education, these principles have been integrated into curricula in multiple ways, including forming a curricular foundational framework (Jeffries, 2005; Reime et al., 2008), bolstering diversity of learning styles (Thompson & Crutchlow, 1993), preparing focused learning modules/methods (Jeffries, 2006), developing simulation frameworks (Reese et al., 2010; Schlairet & Pollock, 2010), and in measurement (Kardong-Edgren et al., 2008). Most recently, the constructs that support the Chickering and Gamson (1987) principles were found as the emerging themes from learners' course evaluation feedback (Taylor et al., 2020).

Chickering and Gamson (1987) provided the theoretical underpinning to the first simulation framework that later became a mid-range theory, NLN Jeffries Simulation theory (Jeffries et al., 2015). Simulation is regarded as a robust active teaching-learning strategy and has proliferated in its use across nursing education (Smiley, 2019). It is well recognized that the debriefing that follows a simulation scenario is the phase of simulation-based education when learners make sense of the experience. Debriefing encompasses many of Chickering and Gamson's (1987) principles for best teaching practices as previously outlined. Because of the significance of this debriefing dialogue to deeper learning, many nursing programs have embraced and applied the constructs of debriefing beyond simulation and across many curricular learning activities. Attributes that must be present in debriefing were identified by Dreifuerst (2009) as reflection, emotional release, feedback, summative evaluation, and integration of new knowledge (Dreifuerst, 2009). It is the reflective style of a debriefing dialogue that guides learners to examine and evaluate their thinking that occurred during their learning experience. In this reflective dialogue, learners can safely discuss the emotions felt during a learning experience and can also receive feedback in a safe space as they integrate new knowledge into their existing frameworks.

An essential component of a rich debriefing conversation is the learner's perception of a psychologically safe learning environment (Rudolph et al., 2007). Psychological safety is defined as an environment in which an individual feels they can take interpersonal risks without fear of shame, humiliation, and belittlement (Edmondson, 1999). As these good teaching principles are integrated into debriefing practices, and debriefing is optimized in the presence of psychological safety, it stands to reason that psychological safety is an additional element of good teaching practices. If learners do not feel safe to share their thoughts, reflective dialogue will feel restrictive, thereby limiting the learning potential.

The defining attributes of debriefing (Dreifuerst, 2009) are synergistic with the guiding principles of best practice in education (Chickering & Gamson, 1987), collectively describing a teaching and learning environment that fosters active learning and the development of reflective thinking. As simulation educators and researchers build the evidence for the positive outcomes of debriefing, this evidence of deep learning from debriefing pedagogy can be applied to intentionally designed active learning experiences across the curriculum. Deeper levels of learning are possible when an educator facilitates collaborative discussions, with a focus on guiding learners' reflection as they integrate feedback to and from their peers.

The NLN published a Vision Statement in 2015 entitled Debriefing Across the Curriculum (NLN, 2015b). The focus of this Vision Statement (2015b) supported integrating debriefing across the curriculum – not just in simulation – as a potential to transform nursing education. Today, more than ever, this Vision Statement holds great promise in providing guidance to educators as they guide learners to be the reflective practitioners necessary in today's health care system. In this work, educators need guidance in evaluating the teaching practices used across the curriculum against the theoretical underpinnings guiding best practice standards.

ESTABLISHING A BASELINE BENCHMARK TO ASSESS TEACHING AND LEARNING ACROSS THE CURRICULUM

As previously stated, the defining attributes of debriefing (Dreifuerst, 2009) are synergistic with the guiding principles of best practice in education (Chickering & Gamson, 1987). Together, they offer guidance; when melded, the impact increases. The principles of encouraging contact between educators and learners, developing reciprocity and cooperation among learners, using active learning techniques, giving prompt feedback, emphasizing time on task, communicating high expectations, and respecting diverse talents and ways of learning, all encompassed in teaching and learning strategies that enhance reflective and metacognitive thinking, are tenets upon which assessing educational practices may be benchmarked. The NLN Educational Practices in Simulation Scale (EPSS), grounded in the seven principles, was used in the research work of Jeffries and colleagues from 2003 to 2006 to evaluate the outcomes of educational practices, such as simulation (Jeffries & Rizzolo, 2006).

The NLN EPSS (now referred to as the NLN EPQ [Educational Practices Questionnaire]) is a 32-item instrument using a five-point Likert scale intended to assess learner and educator perceptions of the presence and importance of four of Chickering and Gamson's (1987) seven best educational practices in instructor-developed simulation (Jeffries & Rizzolo, 2006). The items of the original EPQ are categorized into the subscales of *active learning, collaboration, diverse ways of learning*, and *high expectations*. These subscales represent four elements of the seven guiding principles of Chickering and Gamson (1987) that describe quality teaching and learning across higher education.

Psychometric testing demonstrated a high level of internal consistency (Cronbach's alpha = 0.95) for the overall scale, as well as discrimination scores ranging from 75 to 95 percent (Franklin et al., 2014).

Although the EPQ was intended for use in assessing simulation learning activities, Chickering and Gamson's (1987) principles are not limited to simulation. If simulation as an active teaching-learning strategy undergoes evaluation against benchmark practices, all teaching and learning activities likewise require assessment against a benchmark. However, there is little evidence available to provide explicit feedback on educator teaching practices in a standardized manner.

With evidence of both reliability and validity as a tool for use in simulation, the EPQ provides a baseline instrument which can be expanded for use in assessing teaching and learning across the curriculum using all seven of the best educational practices (Chickering & Gamson, 1987) and the incorporation of reflection. Using seminal benchmark principles, such as those of Chickering and Gamson (1987), to assess the teaching practices of educators in a standardized, reliable way will not only serve to strengthen and improve teaching and learning but will also advance the science of nursing education.

The EPQ, with permission from the NLN, was recently revised to not only address the best educational practices in simulation, but to reach beyond and examine how this reliable instrument, which measures educational best practices in one setting, could be expanded upon to measure educational best practices across educational settings. After a thorough review of the literature on Chickering and Gamson's (1987) seven principles of good teaching practices and the concept of debriefing and its principles, the instrument was revised to add statements that were inclusive of all seven of these principles and the use of reflective teaching practices. The newly revised instrument is entitled NLN Educational Practices Questionnaire-Curriculum (EPQ-C) to reflect the intended purpose of the instrument: to evaluate the use of best practices in teaching and learning across all educational environments. A rigorous process of expert review of the items was conducted to determine the best way to represent the seven principles in the instrument, in a way that could help educators assess and evaluate the teaching-learning experience to improve their teaching. The newly revised instrument has 44 items with an overall CVI of 90. See Box 5.1 for a cross-section of items representing each of Chickering and Gamson's seven principles.

There are a total of 44 items; however, like the original EPQ, each item is rated on two different Likert-type scales. The first 22 items are rated by learners using a 5-point scale about their perceived disagreement or agreement with learning experience; then, the same 22 items are rated by learners on a 5-point Likert-type scale rating their perception of the importance of the item to their learning experience, yielding a possible total score for both parts of 44 to 220.

SUMMARY

The NLN continues to support nurse educators as they strive to create educational experiences that are evidence-based and inclusive of the diverse learners of today. For more than a decade, the NLN has promoted simulation as a teaching methodology to

> **BOX 5.1**
>
> ## Sample Items from Each Category of the EPQ-C
>
> **Student-Faculty Interaction**
> My instructor responded to my needs during the learning experience.
>
> **Collaborative Learning**
> I had the opportunity to discuss the ideas and concepts with other learners during the learning experience.
>
> **Active Learning**
> I had the opportunity to learn how to apply course concepts to future real-life experiences.
>
> **Feedback**
> I received feedback from the instructor about my thinking during the learning experience.
>
> **Time on Task**
> In the given time frame for the learning experience, there were enough moments to incorporate the material in ways that helped me apply it to my learning.
>
> **High Expectations**
> The instructor provided an environment for learning that encouraged me to challenge my own thinking and abilities.
>
> **Diverse Learning**
> The instructor individualized the learning experience to meet my particular needs.

Reprinted with permission from the National League for Nursing.

prepare nurses for practice across the continuum of care in today's complex health care environment. That experience, reinforced by the League's mission and core values, furnishes a strong foundation to address the challenges and opportunities arising in higher education today. Preparing reflective practitioners who are able to use complex data to solve clinical problems requires nurse educators to examine biases and assumptions about traditional education. As new approaches to teaching and learning are adopted, assessment of those practices is vital. As another step in bringing the NLN Vision Statement to life, the EPQ-C provides educators with an assessment tool to guide this.

References

Alexander, B., Ashford-Rowe, K., Barajas-Murph, N., Dobbin, G., Knott, J., McCormack, M., Pomerantz, J., Seilhamer, R., & Weber, N. (2019). Horizon Report 2019 Higher Education Edition. EDU19. https://www.learntechlib.org/p/208644/

Argawal, P. K. (2019). Retrieval practice and Bloom's Taxonomy: Do students need fact knowledge before higher order learning? *Journal of Educational Psychology*, *111*(2), 189–209. https://doi.org/10.1037/edu0000282

Cardoza, M. P. (2011). Neuroscience and simulation: An evolving theory of brain-based education. *Clinical Simulation in Nursing, 7*(6), e205–e208. https://doi.org/10.1016/j.ecns.2011.08.004

Chickering, A. W., & Gamson, Z. F. (1987). Seven principles for practices in undergraduate education. *Journal of Nursing Education, 39*(2), 3–6.

Cowperthwait, A. (2020). NLN/Jeffries Simulation Framework for simulated participant methodology. *Clinical Simulation in Nursing, 42*, 12–21. https://doi.org/10.1016/j.ecns.2019.12.009

Doyle, T., & Zakrajsek, T. (2019). *The new science of learning: How to learn in harmony with your brain* (2nd ed.). Stylus Publishing. https://lccn.loc.gov/2018022978

Dreifuerst, K. T. (2009). The essentials of debriefing in simulation learning: A concept analysis. *Nursing Education Perspectives, 30*(2), 109–114.

Edmondson, A. (1999). Psychological safety and learning behavior in work teams. *Administrative Science Quarterly, 44*(2), 350–383. http://www.jstor.org/stable/2666999

Forneris, S. G., & Fey, M. (Eds.). (2020). *Critical conversations (Volume 2): From monologue to dialogue.* National League for Nursing. ISBN/ISSN:9781975168568

Franklin, A., Burns, P., & Lee, C. (2014). Psychometric testing on the NLN Student Satisfaction and Self-Confidence in Learning, Simulation Design Scale, and Educational Practices Questionnaire using a sample of pre-licensure novice students. *Nurse Education Today, 34*, 1298–1304. https://dx.doi.org/10.1016/j.nedt.2014.06.011

INACSL Board of Directors. (2011). Standards of Best Practice: Simulation^{SM}. *Clinical Simulation in Nursing, 7*(4S), s1–s19. https://doi.org/10.1016/j.ecns.2011.05.005

INACSL Standards Committee. (2016). INACSL Standards of Best Practice: Simulation^{SM}. *Clinical Simulation in Nursing, 12*, S5–S50. https://doi.org/10.1016/j.ecns.2016.09.009

Jeffries, P. R. (2005). A framework for designing, implementing, and evaluating simulations used as teaching strategies in nursing. *Nursing Education Perspectives, 26*(2), 96–103.

Jeffries, P. R. (2006). Guest editor: Developing evidenced-based teaching strategies and practices when using simulation. *Clinical Simulation in Nursing, 2*(1), E1–E2. https://doi.org/10.1016/j.ecns.2009.05.014

Jeffries, P. R., & Rizzolo, M. A. (2006). Summary report: Designing and implementing models for the innovative use of simulation to teach nursing care of ill adults and children: A national, multi-site, multi-method study. National League for Nursing. http://www.nln.org/docs/default-source/professional-development-programs/read-the-nln-laerdal-project-summary-report-pdf.pdf?sfvrsn=0

Jeffries, P. R., Rodgers, B., & Adamson, K. (2015). NLN Jeffries Simulation theory: Brief narrative description. *Nursing Education Perspectives, 36*(5), 292–293. https://doi.org/10.1097/00024776-201509000-00004

Jones, I., & Alinier, G. (2015). Supporting students' learning experiences through a pocket size cue card designed around a reflective Simulation Framework. *Clinical Simulation in Nursing, 11*(7), 325–334. https://doi.org/10.1016/j.ecns.2015.04.004

Kardong-Edgren, Suzan E., Starkweather, Angela Renee, and Ward, Linda D. "The Integration of Simulation into a Clinical Foundations of Nursing Course: Student and Faculty Perspectives." *International Journal of Nursing Education Scholarship*, vol. 5, no. 1, 2008, pp. 1–16. https://doi.org/10.2202/1548-923X.1603

National Academy of Medicine. (2020). The future of nursing: 2020–2030. Retrieved from https://nam.edu/publications/the-future-of-nursing-2020-2030/

National League for Nursing. (2015a). A vision for teaching with simulation. Retrieved from http://www.nln.org/docs/default-source/about/nln-vision-series-(position-statements)/vision-statement-a-vision-for-teaching-with-simulation.pdf?sfvrsn=2

National League for Nursing. (2015b). Debriefing across the curriculum. Retrieved from http://www.nln.org/docs/default-source/about/nln-vision-series-(position-statements)/

nln-vision-debriefing-across-the-curriculum
.pdf?sfvrsn=0

Nestel, D., & Bearman, M. (2015). Theory and simulation-based education: Definitions, worldviews and applications. *Clinical Simulation in Nursing, 11*(8), 349–354. https://doi.org/10.1016/j.ecns.2015.05.013

Pan, S. C., & Rickard, T. C. (2018). Transfer of test-enhanced learning: Meta-analytic review and synthesis. *Psychological Bulletin, 144*(7), 710–756. https://doi.org/10.1037/bul0000151

Reese, C. E., Jeffries, P. R., & Engum, S. A. (2010). Learning together: Using simulations to develop nursing and medical student collaboration. *Nursing Education Perspectives, 31*(1), 33–37.

Reime, M. H., Harris, A., Aksnes, J., & Mikkelsen, J. (2008). The most successful method in teaching nursing students infection control – E-learning or lecture? *Nurse Education Today, 28*(7), 798–806. https://doi.org/10.1016/j.nedt.2008.03.005

Rudolph, J. W., Simon, R., Rivard, P., Dufresne, R. L., & Raemer, D. B. (2007). Debriefing with good judgment: Combining rigorous feedback with genuine inquiry. *Anesthesiology Clinics, 25*(2), 361–376. https://doi.org/10.1016/j.anclin.2007.03.007

Schlairet, M. C., & Pollock, J. W. (2010). Equivalence testing of traditional and simulated clinical experiences: Undergraduate nursing students' knowledge acquisition. *Journal of Nursing Education, 49*(1), 43–47. https://doi.org/10.3928/01484834-20090918-08

Smiley, R. A. (2019). Survey of simulation use in prelicensure nursing programs: Changes and advancements. *Journal of Nursing Regulation, 9*(4), 48–61. https://doi.org/10.1016/S2155-8256(19)30016-X

Taylor, R. L., Knorr, K., Ogrodnik, M., & Sinclair, P. (2020). Seven principles for good practice in midterm student feedback. *International Journal for Academic Development, 25*(4), 350–362. https://doi.org/10.1080/1360144X.2020.1762086

Thompson, C., & Crutchlow, E. (1993). Learning style research: A critical review of the literature and implications for nursing education. *Journal of Professional Nursing, 9*(1), 34–40. https://doi.org/10.1016/8755-7223(93)90084-p

Waxman, K. T., Bowler, F., Forneris, S. G., Kardong-Edgren, S., & Rizzolo, M. A. (2019). Simulation as a nursing education disrupter. *Nursing Administration Quarterly, 43*(4), 300–305. https://doi.org/10.1097/NAQ.0000000000000369

Weidman, J., & Baker, K. (2015). The cognitive science of learning: Concepts and strategies for the educator and learner. *Neuroscience in Anesthesiology and Perioperative Medicine, 121*(6), 1586–1599. https://doi.org/10.1213/ANE.0000000000000890

6

Future Research and Next Steps

Beth Rodgers, PhD, RN, FAAN
Katie Anne Haerling (Adamson), PhD, RN, CHSE
Pamela R. Jeffries, PhD, RN, FAAN, ANEF

INTRODUCTION

The 2016 systematic review of the literature completed as part of the development of the National League for Nursing (NLN) Jeffries Simulation theory enabled identification of recurring themes, gaps, and key issues, as well as insight into what constituted best practices and priorities for future simulation research. While completing that work, the authors simultaneously identified priority areas for future research. In this chapter, the authors briefly highlight the earlier (2016) findings for research and how those have evolved (see Table 6.1), which provides some historical perspective on the state of simulation research. Following a brief review of earlier research, specific themes and emerging areas for research are provided to guide future research and development of simulation science (see Table 6.2). Although many of the priorities identified in the 2016 publication remain, there has been an obvious shift in some aspects of simulation research.

PRIOR THEMES AND ADVANCES IN SIMULATION RESEARCH

The earlier review, published in the 2016 monograph (Jeffries, 2016), revealed the state of simulation overall as a still emerging modality for education. Early research in simulation in nursing generally was focused on a broad view of simulation: what could be accomplished with simulation, how simulation could be used to enhance student educational experiences, how to provide simulation experiences, and some basic ideas about how to structure simulated clinical work and evaluate student participation and learning. A common theme in this research also included economic models for simulation along with support for the cost-effectiveness of simulation. Although numerous studies have shown that simulation was a successful teaching modality, questions persist on how much, and how, to implement to ensure quality outcomes. A significant factor in the creation of this situation was the development of simulation laboratories

65

TABLE 6.1

Themes for Research in Simulation: 2016 Review

Theme Emerged	Topic
Cost effectiveness/economic model	Is simulation cost-effective and how can educational practices and simulation design characteristics be manipulated to optimize the cost-effectiveness equation (Kennedy et al., 2013; Weaver, 2011)?
Improved outcomes – the efficacy of simulation	Do gains from simulation last and do they translate into improved outcomes? There is a need for longitudinal data about the efficacy of simulation and skill decay (Finan et al., 2012; McGaghie, 2008; Weaver, 2011; Yeung et al., 2013).
	There is a need for improved measurement practices and research designs, including better interpretations of statistical and clinical significance of findings (Harder, 2010; LeFlore et al., 2012; McGaghie, 2008; Yeung et al., 2013; Yuan et al., 2012).
Self-efficacy/self-confidence, competence/performance, and so on, and the relationships of these constructs	There is a need to further investigate the relationships between confidence/self-efficacy, knowledge gains, competence/performance, and patient outcomes (Burke, 2010; Dobbs et al., 2006; Hauber et al., 2010; McGaghie, 2008; Rosen et al., 2012; Tiffen et al., 2011; Wilson & Hagler, 2012).
Best educational practices – defining and describing	Determining what are "good" educational practices and whether simulation or other educational practices make simulation effective (Hallenbeck, 2012). Determining which scenarios are more effective: simple or complex (Guhde, 2011; Parker & Myrick, 2012). Determining which lab is more effective: virtual or skill (Durmaz et al., 2012; Ravert, 2002).
Fidelity	Can the notion of fidelity be clarified and standardized so that evidence regarding best practices related to fidelity can be identified?

TABLE 6.2

Emerging, New Themes for Research Found in the 2021 Systematic Review

Continuing and Emerging Themes	Topics
Best educational practices	Research examining "good" or "best" educational practices has exploded. Specific issues identified as part of the 2021 review include: • What are best practices when simulation is used to teach concepts such as cultural sensitivity, cultural competency, and cultural humility? Do these activities translate into improved patient care and outcomes (Foronda et al., 2018)? • What is the comparative effectiveness of various strategies (and combinations of strategies) for pre-briefing and debriefing simulation activities in terms of learning, behavior, and outcomes (Ali et al., 2018; Dileone et al., 2020; McDermott, 2020; Tyerman et al., 2019; Wilbanks et al., 2020)?

(*continued*)

	• What are best practices for optimizing learning outcomes for participants in the observer role of simulation (Rogers et al., 2020)?
Fidelity	Now that fidelity has been well defined (INACSL, 2016; Lioce et al., 2020), some investigators have begun to examine specific dimensions of fidelity (Lavoie et al., 2020; Mills et al., 2016).
Use of virtual simulations: when, where, how?	The importance of the question has only grown. While additional evidence has emerged to address this question, new technologies and the explosion in the use of virtual technologies have expanded the question to include a variety of simulation modalities (Coyne, 2021; Haerling, 2018).
Improved outcomes, specifically: Efficacy of simulation Self-efficacy/self-confidence, competence/performance, and so on, and the relationships of these constructs	The evidence increasingly demonstrates that gains realized in simulation translate to patient care and patient outcomes, but more research is needed (Bruce et al., 2019; Seaton et al., 2019). Research has moved away from an over-reliance on self-confidence and satisfaction as measures of success in simulation and more studies are using higher levels of evaluation including patient outcomes (Seaton et al., 2019). To underscore the importance of moving away from self-confidence as a measure of simulation effectiveness, Donohue et al. (2020) demonstrated that "self-reported efficacy had no correlation to clinical skills in neonatal resuscitation; participants both overestimated and underestimated their clinical proficiency" (p. 377).
Nurse practitioner education and the use of simulations	How do simulation-based experiences used in nurse practitioner education affect learning, behavior, and patient outcomes (Warren et al., 2016)?
Adaptive technologies to be harnessed in the simulation environment to improve performance	How can adaptive technologies be harnessed within the simulation environment to improve both individual and collective performance (Lineberry et al., 2018)?
Benefits and optimization of virtual simulations	How can the benefits of virtual simulation be optimized? For example, Foronda et al. (2020) point out the need for research on virtual simulation compared to manikin-based simulation, effects of virtual simulation throughout the curriculum, and delivery of virtual simulation in regard to amount and timing of the simulation experiences (p. 52).
Guidelines and instructional design features in developing health care simulations	The Reporting Guidelines for Healthcare Simulation Research (Cheng et al., 2016) and subsequent call for inclusion of instructional design features to be included in health care simulation research reports (Salas, 2016) address this need but have not resolved the issue. One topic, specifically relevant to the NLN Jeffries Simulation theory, related to what constitutes the "Simulation Experience." The INACSL Standards indicate the simulation-based experience is "[a] broad array of structured activities that represent actual or potential situations in education, practice, and research" (p. S45), but then goes on to say the pre-brief is "an information or orientation session immediately prior to the start of a simulation-based experience." Much of the research implies the simulation experience includes all activities from pre-brief through debrief, but this is not stated explicitly.

and centers but a lack of clear guidance for full utilization of those resources. From that beginning focus on whether or not simulation "works," research has grown to look more specifically at components of simulation, how to construct and deliver quality simulation, and how to maximize the learning that takes place in simulation.

SUMMARY AND FUTURE DIRECTIONS

This review highlights some of the continuing and emerging trends in research evident in the literature. Looking specifically at existing research will reveal areas of greatest activity, which is enlightening in understanding the state of simulation science overall. There are other areas that are in need of exploration based on emerging priorities and also some obvious gaps in the literature. In spite of the amount of research that has been done on simulation, there is a need for greater attention to theory-driven research to advance simulation theory. The topic of simulation delivery, particularly the facilitator role and ways to guide simulation activity for students, has not been explored well. People working in the area of simulation can benefit from research-based insight into how to deliver, guide, and facilitate quality simulation. While there has been a great deal of attention paid to debriefing as a focus of learning, there are other opportunities for active learning throughout simulation experiences that are not examined well in the existing literature. Research also is needed to look at simulation as a whole, including an expanded emphasis on the entire process of pre-briefing through debriefing and closure, in examining design. Theory-driven research is especially needed to support development in a cohesive manner with clear concepts and language that facilitate sharing and synthesis of knowledge.

The field of simulation is exciting and developing rapidly. One focus of this monograph overall has been to provide guidance for best practices and for the discovery of new knowledge and practices in this clinical area. In this chapter, trends and areas of ongoing research emphasis have been described briefly to bring attention to the research base and aspects of simulation that are particularly in need of development. The NLN Jeffries Simulation theory serves to articulate the phenomenon and the relationships among aspects of simulation to guide practice and further research. The challenge is to continue use and evaluation of the theory in a variety of settings and for new findings to be advanced in development of the theory and the science of simulation.

References

Ali, A. A., & Musallam, E. (2018, March). Debriefing quality evaluation in nursing simulation-based education: An integrative review. *Clinical Simulation in Nursing, 16*, 15–24. https://doi.org/10.1016/j.ecns.2017.09.009

Bruce, R., Levett-Jones, T., & Courtney-Pratt, H. (2019, October). Transfer of learning from university-based simulation experiences to nursing students' future clinical practice: An exploratory study. *Clinical Simulation in Nursing, 35*(C), 17–24. https://doi.org/10.1016/j.ecns.2019.06.003

Burke, P. M. (2010). A simulation case study from an instructional design framework. *Teaching & Learning in Nursing, 5*(2), 73–77. https://doi.org/10.1016/j.teln.2010.01.003

Cheng, A., Kessler, D., Mackinnon, R., Chang, T. P., Nadkarni, V. M., Hunt, E. A., Duval-Arnould, J., Lin, Y., Cook, D. A., Pusic, M., Hui, J., Moher, D., Egger, M., & Auerbach, M. (2016). Reporting guidelines for health care simulation research: Extensions to the CONSORT and STROBE statements. *Simulation in Healthcare, 11*(4), 238–248. https://doi.org/10.1186/s41077-016-0025-y

Coyne, E., Calleja, P., Forster, E., & Lin, F. (2021). A review of virtual-simulation for assessing healthcare students' clinical competency. *Nurse Education Today, 96*, 104623. doi: 10.1016/j.nedt.2020.104623

Dileone, C., Chyun, D., Diaz, D., & Maruca, A. (2020). An examination of simulation prebriefing in nursing education. *Nursing Education Perspectives*, *41*(6), 345–348. doi: 10.1097/01.NEP.0000000000000689

Dobbs, C., Sweitzer, V., & Jeffries, P. (2006). Testing simulation design features using an insulin management simulation in nursing education. *Clinical Simulation in Nursing*, *2*(1), e17–e22. doi: 10.1016/j.ecns.2009.05.012

Donohue, L. T., Underwood, M. A., & Hoffman, K. R. (2020). Relationship between self-efficacy and performance of simulated neonatal chest compressions and ventilation. *Simulation in Healthcare*, *15*(6), 377–381. doi: 10.1097/SIH.0000000000000446

Durmaz, A., Dicle, A., Cakan, E., & Cakir, S. (2012). Effect of screen-based computer simulation on knowledge and skill in nursing students' learning of preoperative and postoperative care management: A randomized controlled study. *CIN: Computers, Informatics, Nursing*, *30*(4), 196–203. Retrieved from http://search.ebscohost.com/login.aspx?direct=true&db=rzh&AN=2011583355&site=ehost-live

Finan, E., Bismilla, Z., Campbell, C., LeBlanc, V., Jefferies, A., & Whyte, H. E. (2012). Improved procedural performance following a simulation training session may not be transferable to the clinical environment. *Journal of Perinatology*, *32*(7), 539–544. https://doi.org/10.1038/jp.2011.141

Foronda, C. L., Baptiste, D.-L., Pfaff, T., Velez, R., Reinholdt, M., Sanchez, M., & Hudson, K. W. (2018, February). Cultural competency and cultural humility in simulation-based education: An integrative review. *Clinical Simulation in Nursing*, *15*, 42–60. https://doi.org/10.1016/j.ecns.2017.09.006

Foronda, C. L., Fernandez-Burgos, M., Nadeau, C., Kelley, C. N., & Henry, M. N. (2020). Virtual simulation in nursing education: A systematic review spanning 1996 to 2018. *Simulation in Healthcare*, *15*(1), 46–54. doi: 10.1097/SIH.0000000000000411

Guhde, J. (2011). Nursing students' perceptions of the effect on critical thinking, assessment, and learner satisfaction in simple versus complex high-fidelity simulation scenarios. *The Journal of Nursing Education*, *50*(2), 73–78.

Haerling, K. A. (2018). Cost-utility analysis of virtual and mannequin-based simulation. *Simulation in Healthcare*, *13*(1), 1–40. doi: 10.1097/SIH.0000000000000280

Hallenbeck, V. J. (2012). Use of high-fidelity simulation for staff education/development: A systematic review of the literature. *Journal for Nurses in Staff Development*, *28*(6), 260. https://doi.org/10.1097/NND.0b013e31827259c7

Harder, B. N. (2010). Use of simulation in teaching and learning in health sciences: A systematic review. *Journal of Nursing Education*, *49*(1), 23–28. https://doi.org/10.3928/01484834-20090828-08

Hauber, R. P., Cormier, E., & Whyte, I. J. (2010). An exploration of the relationship between knowledge and performance-related variables in high-fidelity simulation: Designing instruction that promotes expertise in practice. *Nursing Education Perspectives*, *31*(4), 242–246. Retrieved from http://search.ebscohost.com/login.aspx?direct=true&db=rzh&AN=2010913909&site=ehost-live

INACSL Standards Committee. (2016, December). INACSL Standards of Best Practice: Simulation©: Simulation glossary. *Clinical Simulation in Nursing*, *12*, S39–S47. https://doi.org/10.1016/j.ecns.2016.09.012

Jeffries, P. R. (2016). *The NLN Jeffries Simulation theory*. Wolters Kluwer.

Kennedy, C. C., Maldonado, F., & Cook, D. A. (2013). Simulation-based bronchoscopy training: Systematic review and meta-analysis. *Chest*, *144*(1), 183–192. https://doi.org/10.1378/chest.12-1786

Lavoie, P., Deschênes, M.-F., Nolin, R., Belisle, M., Blanchet Garneau, A., Boyer, L., Lapierre, A., & Fernandez, N. (2020, May). Beyond technology: A scoping review of features that promote fidelity and authenticity in simulation-based health professional education. *Clinical Simulation in Nursing*, *42*(C), 22–41. https://doi.org/10.1016/j.ecns.2020.02.001

LeFlore, J., Anderson, M., Zielke, M., Nelson, K., Thomas, P., Hardee, G., & John, L. (2012). Can a virtual patient trainer teach student nurses how to save lives — Teaching nursing students about pediatric respiratory diseases. *Simulation in Healthcare, 7*, 10–17. https://doi.org/10.1097/SIH.0b013e31823652de

Lineberry, M., Dev, P., Lane, H. C., & Talbot, T. B. (2018). Learner-adaptive educational technology for simulation in healthcare: Foundations and opportunities. *Simulation in Healthcare, 13*(3S Suppl 1), S21–S27. doi 10.1097/SIH.0000000000000274

Lioce, L. (Ed.), Downing, D., Chang, T. P., Robertson, J. M., Anderson, M., Diaz, D. A., & Spain, A. E. (Assoc. Eds.) and the Terminology and Concepts Working Group. (2020, January). *Healthcare simulation dictionary – Second Edition*. Agency for Healthcare Research and Quality. AHRQ Publication No. 20-0019. https://doi.org/10.23970/simulationv2

McDermott, D. S. (2020, December). Prebriefing: A historical perspective and evolution of a model and strategy (know: do: teach). *Clinical Simulation in Nursing, 49*(C), 40–49. https://doi.org/10.1016/j.ecns.2020.05.005

McGaghie, W. C. (2008). Research opportunities in simulation-based medical education using deliberate practice. *Academic Emergency Medicine, 15*(11), 995–1001. Retrieved from http://search.ebscohost.com/login.aspx?direct=true&db=rzh&AN=2010386653&site=ehost-live

Mills, B. W., Carter, O., Rudd, C., Claxton, L. A., Ross, N. P., & Strobel, N. A. (2016). Effects of low- versus high-fidelity simulations on the cognitive burden and performance of entry-level paramedicine students: A mixed-methods comparison trial using eye-tracking, continuous heart rate, difficulty rating scales, video observation and interviews. *Simulation in Healthcare, 11*(1), 10–18. doi: 10.1097/SIH.0000000000000119

Parker, B. C., & Myrick, F. (2012). The pedagogical ebb and flow of human patient simulation: Empowering through a process of fading support. *Journal of Nursing Education, 51*(7), 365–372. https://doi.org/10.3928/01484834-20120509-01

Ravert, P. (2002). An integrative review of computer-based simulation in the education process. *CIN: Computers, Informatics, Nursing, 20*(5), 203–208. Retrieved from http://search.ebscohost.com/login.aspx?direct=true&db=rzh&AN=2002159431&site=ehost-live

Rogers, B., Baker, K. A., & Franklin, A. E. (2020, December). Learning outcomes of the observer role in nursing simulation: A scoping review. *Clinical Simulation in Nursing, 49*(C), 81–89. https://doi.org/10.1016/j.ecns.2020.06.003

Rosen, M. A., Hunt, E. A., Pronovost, P. J., Federowicz, M. A., & Weaver, S. J. (2012). In situ simulation in continuing education for the health care professions: A systematic review. *Journal of Continuing Education in the Health Professions, 32*(4), 243–254. https://doi.org/10.1002/chp.21152

Salas, E. (2016). Reporting guidelines for health are simulation research: Where is the learning? *Simulation in Healthcare, 11*(4), 249. doi: 10.1097/SIH.0000000000000187

Seaton, P., Levett-Jones, T., Cant, R., Cooper, S., Kelly, M. A., McKenna, L., Ng, L., & Bogossian, F. (2019). Exploring the extent to which simulation-based education addresses contemporary patient safety priorities: A scoping review. *Collegian (Royal College of Nursing, Australia), 26*(1), 194–203. https://doi.org/10.1016/j.colegn.2018.04.006

Tiffen, J., Corbridge, S., Shen, B. C., & Robinson, P. (2011). Patient simulator for teaching heart and lung assessment skills to advanced practice nursing students. *Clinical Simulation in Nursing, 7*(3), e91–e97. https://doi.org/10.1016/j.ecns.2009.10.003

Tyerman, J., Luctkar-Flude, M., Graham, L., Coffey, S., & Olsen-Lynch, E. (2019, February). A systematic review of health care presimulation preparation and briefing effectiveness. *Clinical Simulation in Nursing, 27*(C), 12–25. https://doi.org/10.1016/j.ecns.2018.11.002

Warren, J. N., Luctkar-Flude, M., Godfrey, C., & Lukewich, J. (2016). A systematic review of the effectiveness of simulation-based education on satisfaction and learning outcomes in nurse practitioner programs. *Nurse Education Today, 46*, 99–108. doi: 10.1016/j.nedt.2016.08.023

Weaver, A. (2011). High-fidelity patient simulation in nursing education: An integrative review. *Nursing Education Perspectives*, *32*(1), 37–40. https://doi.org/10.5480/1536-5026-32.1.37

Wilbanks, B. A., McMullan, S., Watts, P. I., White, T., & Moss, J. (2020, May). Comparison of videofacilitated reflective practice and faculty-led debriefings. *Clinical Simulation in Nursing*, *42*(C), 1–7. https://doi.org/10.1016/j.ecns.2019.12.007

Wilson, R. D., & Hagler, D. (2012). Through the lens of instructional design: Appraisal of the Jeffries/National League for Nursing Simulation Framework for use in acute care. *Journal of Continuing Education in Nursing*, *43*(9), 428–432. https://doi.org/10.3928/00220124-20120615-27

Yeung, E., Dubrowski, A., & Carnahan, H. (2013). Simulation-augmented education in the rehabilitation professions: A scoping review. *International Journal of Therapy & Rehabilitation*, *20*(5), 228–236. Retrieved from http://search.ebscohost.com/login.aspx?direct=true&db=rzh&AN=2012127287&site=ehost-live

Yuan, H. B., Williams, B. A., & Fang, J. B. (2012). The contribution of high-fidelity simulation to nursing students' confidence and competence: A systematic review. *International Nursing Review*, *59*(1), 26–33. https://doi.org/10.1111/j.1466-7657.2011.00964.x